# HEART SOUNDS
## AND MURMURS

THIRD EDITION

# HEART SOUNDS AND MURMURS

## A PRACTICAL GUIDE

**BARBARA ERICKSON, PhD, RN, CCRN**
Critical Care Clinical Nurse
Specialist/Case Manager
Western Reserve Care System
Youngstown, Ohio

with 54 illustrations

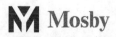
Mosby

St. Louis  Baltimore  Boston  Carlsbad  Chicago  Naples  New York  Philadelphia  Portland
London  Madrid  Mexico City  Singapore  Sydney  Tokyo  Toronto  Wiesbaden

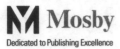

**Mosby**
Dedicated to Publishing Excellence

A Times Mirror
Company

*Vice President and Publisher:* Nancy Coon
*Editor:* Barry Bowlus
*Developmental Editor:* Cynthia Anderson
*Project Manager:* Deborah L. Vogel
*Production Editor:* Sarah E. Fike
*Manufacturing Supervisor:* Linda Ierardi

**THIRD EDITION**
**Copyright © 1997 by Mosby-Year Book, Inc.**

Previous editions copyrighted 1987, 1991

Printed in the United States of America
Composition by Clarinda Company
Lithography/color film by Clarinda Company
Printing/binding by Plus Communications

Mosby-Year Book, Inc.
11830 Westline Industrial Drive
St. Louis, Missouri 63146

**Library of Congress Cataloging in Publication Data**
Erickson, Barbara.
   Heart sounds and murmurs : a practical guide / Barbara Erickson. –
– 3rd ed.
      p.     cm.
   Includes bibliographical references and index.
   ISBN 0-8151-3146-1
   1. Heart—Sounds.   2. Heart—Diseases—Diagnosis.  I. Title.
   [DNLM:  1. Heart Auscultation—programmed instruction.  WG 18.2
E68h 1996]
   RC683.5.A9E73   1996
   616.1'2—dc20
   DNLM/DLC
for Library of Congress                         96-29333
                                                        CIP

98 99 00 / 9 8 7 6 5 4 3 2

To
Leonard P. Caccamo, MD, FACP, FACC
*Mentor, Friend, and Inspiration*
*and*
Frank C. Tiberio, MD
*Clinician and Auscultator Extraordinaire*

# PREFACE

Cardiac auscultation is coming into prominence again and is being recognized as an important diagnostic tool alongside more modern technologies such as scans, echos, and Doppler scans. The information derived from a properly used stethoscope is invaluable. In the hands of an individual prepared to use it, the stethoscope is a cost-effective, cost-containing invaluable instrument.

Proficiency in cardiac auscultation does not come with the acquisition of a quality stethoscope. The most important prerequisite for effective auscultation is a prepared mind. The clinician should be aware of the dynamics of the cardiac cycle during auscultation and integrate each heart sound and murmur heard with a corresponding hemodynamic effect.

The third edition of this book expands on the information and interpretations found in the earlier editions to include sounds heard when mechanical or biological values in various positions are ausculated. In addition, sounds generated by an intraaortic balloon pump, pacemaker, sternal click, and intracardiac myxomas are discussed.

This program is intended for the beginning auscultator who wishes to learn the basics of listening to and interpreting heart sounds. The more advanced auscultator may find the program helpful as a review of the basics of listening to and interpreting heart sounds.

The format used is one that has proven successful to the author over many years of teaching heart sounds. Basic information in the text is accompanied by an audio program. By first reading the text and then listening to the audio program, the learner should have the essential information necessary to understand and recognize the normal heart sounds and the most common abnormal sounds.

To become clinically proficient in recognizing heart sounds, the learner must continually listen to as many hearts as possible. However good the reproduction of heart sounds on the audio program may be, the program can never replace the experience of listening to actual heart sounds. Please remember that the sounds on the audio program have been distinctly simulated to facilitate learning. Sounds from real hearts will be similar but never heard as clearly as those on the audio program.

The audio program was made with sounds from a real heart and sounds from a heart sound simulator, using studio recording equipment.

Barbara Erickson

# INSTRUCTIONS FOR USE

**The learner is advised to:**

1. Read the basic information found in the text regarding the sound.
2. Listen to the sound on the accompanying audio program, which should be repeatedly listened to until the learner is able to discern the sound being described. Before proceeding to the next section the learner must understand and *identify* each sound being described.
3. Listen to the audio program with a stethoscope placed about 4 inches from the speaker. For best results, the audio program should be played on quality equipment. The better the sound transmission of the equipment, the better the learner will be able to hear subtle differences on the heart sound audio program.
4. Listen to real hearts. Repeatedly practice listening to heart sounds to gain proficiency and expertise.
5. Test your knowledge of the content of each chapter by:
   a. Comparing behavioral objectives given at the beginning of each chapter to your abilities on completing the chapter.
   b. Answering self-learning questions at the end of each chapter, and checking your answers against those in the answer key.
   c. Listening to the "unknowns" on the audio program at the end of each chapter, and checking your answers against those in the answer key.
6. Refer to the audio program when the symbol ❖ appears in the margin.

# CONTENTS

**Chapter 5**

**Chapter 6**

# CHAPTER 1

## Introduction

**LEARNING OBJECTIVES**

After reading this chapter and answering the self-learning questions at the end of the chapter, the learner will be able to do the following:

1. Identify the requirements for adequate cardiac auscultation
2. Differentiate between the use of the bell and diaphragm chestpiece of a stethoscope
3. Identify two basic mechanisms of cardiac sound production
4. Identify the four basic characteristics of sound
5. Differentiate between sounds of high frequency and low frequency
6. Identify three factors that enter into the transmission of sounds
7. Choose the appropriate area on the chest for auscultation of a selected sound
8. Differentiate between ventricular systole, ventricular diastole, and atrial systole
9. Identify the relationship of cardiac sounds to the cardiac cycle
10. Chart heart sounds using the one-through-six classification scale

## HISTORY

The language of the heart, discerned by cardiac auscultation, is a universal medical language. I was dramatically made aware of this while visiting China. Communications needing no interpretation were those of heart sounds, electrocardiograms, and music. By becoming skillful in listening to and interpreting the language of the heart, you also may join a long line of notable semiologists.

Direct auscultation of the heart was known to Hippocrates (460-377 BC), who may have used heart sounds for diagnostic purposes. William Harvey (1578-1657) seems to have been the first to make specific reference to heart sounds. The use of the ear without mechanical aid was the accepted method of listening to the heart until 1816, when René Laënnec invented the first stethoscope. Laënnec (1781-1826), by discovering and perfecting the acoustic trumpet, became known as the "Father of Auscultation." Laënnec named his auscultatory instrument a "stethoscope" from the Greek word meaning "the spy of the chest." His original instrument, which was a hollow wooden cylinder, has been repeatedly revised. These revisions have continued to the present, making available a great variety of quality stethoscopes.

However perfect the instrument of auscultation, the interpretation of the sounds is still of the essence. Although Laënnec devoted his life to the semiology of cardiac auscultation, it was a Czech doctor, Joseph Skoda (1805-1881), who first described the cardiac sounds and murmurs. He pinpointed their locations and defined the clinical auscultatory signs that have allowed the diagnosis of cardiac pathology via auscultation. The learner is advised to mimic Skoda and become proficient in pinpointing the locations of cardiac sounds and murmurs to arrive at a clinical interpretation of their meaning.

## REQUIREMENTS FOR AUSCULTATION

Auscultation must not be performed as an isolated event. The total cardiovascular physical examination includes five important parts: (1) examination of the arterial pulse and blood pressure, (2) inspection of the jugular venous pulse, (3) inspection of the precordium, (4) palpation of the precordium, and (5) auscultation. Each of these parts is important, although only auscultation will be discussed in this book.

One of the first things to consider when undertaking auscultation of the heart is the necessity to do the following:

1. **Use a quiet, well-lit, warm room.** To facilitate hearing the heart sounds, ambient noise in the room should be eliminated as much as possible. This means that room doors are closed and equipment such as radios and televisions are turned off and conversations stopped.

Unfortunately a quiet room may be one of the hardest elements to achieve. The room needs to be well lit so that the inspection aspect of cardiac examination may be done. Many of the heart sounds can be seen and felt as well as heard. A warm room helps keep the patient from shivering and thus causing extraneous sounds underneath the chestpiece of the stethoscope.

2. **Have the patient properly disrobed.** The stethoscope should always be placed in direct contact with the chest wall. Most abnormal sounds cannot be heard through clothing because they are lower in frequency and softer than normal heart sounds. Also, listening through clothing will produce sound distortions caused by the stethoscope rubbing against the clothing.

3. **Examine the patient in three positions—supine, sitting, and left lateral recumbent** (Fig. 1-1). Listening in various positions will bring out certain heart sounds, especially some abnormal ones. For instance, the third heart sound ($S_3$) may be brought out by having the patient turn to the left lateral recumbent position.

4. **Examine the patient from his or her right side.** Being on the patient's right side forces the examiner to reach across the chest to listen to the heart. This stretches out the tubing of the stethoscope and decreases the likelihood of extraneous sounds caused by the tubing hitting objects (e.g., chest wall, side rails).

5. **Use a stethoscope with a bell and diaphragm chestpiece or one with characteristics of both bell and diaphragm.** Traditionally a stethoscope with both a bell and a diaphragm was essential for complete cardiac auscultation. However, recent technology has provided a stethoscope with only one chestpiece capable of differentiating low-frequency from high-frequency sounds, depending on the pressure applied to the chestpiece. When the chestpiece is used with light

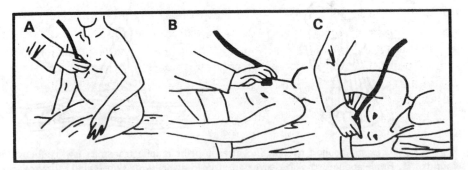

**Fig. I-I.** Basic positions for cardiac auscultation. **A,** sitting; **B,** supine; **C,** left lateral recumbent. (Reproduced with permission from L. Caccamo and B. Erickson, *Cardiac auscultation,* Youngstown, Ohio: St. Elizabeth Hospital Medical Center, 1975.)

pressure, the low-frequency sounds dominate; used with firm pressure the high-frequency sounds are accentuated. Regardless of the technical advances, the traditional principles still apply and therefore will continue to be used in this book.

a. **Using the bell**

When the bell is held *lightly* (leaving no after-imprint on the chest), it picks up *low-frequency* sounds.

Pressure on the bell causes the skin to be pulled tautly over the bottom of the bell, changing the bell to a diaphragm (Fig. 1-2).

b. **Using the diaphragm**

When the diaphragm is applied *firmly* (leaving an after-imprint) it picks up *high-frequency* sounds.

c. **Differentiating frequencies**

The frequency of a sound is readily identified by noting with which chestpiece of the stethoscope the sound is heard best. A sound heard best, or only heard, with the **bell held lightly is of low frequency.** A sound best heard with the **bell applied firmly, or with a diaphragm, is of high frequency.** This simple maneuver of listening to a sound with the bell held lightly and then applied firmly permits you to determine the frequency of the sound to which you are listening. **This is an important point to remember.**

6. **Listen to each area of auscultation.** Listen to each of the following areas, using first the diaphragm and then the bell (Fig. 1-3).

a. Left lateral sternal border (also known as lower left sternal border [LLSB]): This is the fourth intercostal space (4 ICS) to the left of the sternum. Sounds from the tricuspid valve and right heart are heard best.

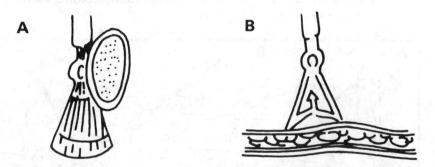

**Fig. 1-2.   A,** *Lightly* applied to skin (no after-imprint is left) transmits *low-frequency* sounds. **B,** *Firmly* applied to skin (leaves an after-imprint) with skin pulled tautly over the bottom of the bell changes it into a diaphragm and transmits *high-frequency* sounds. (Modified with permission from L. Caccamo and B. Erickson, *Cardiac auscultation,* Youngstown, Ohio: St. Elizabeth Hospital Medical Center, 1975.)

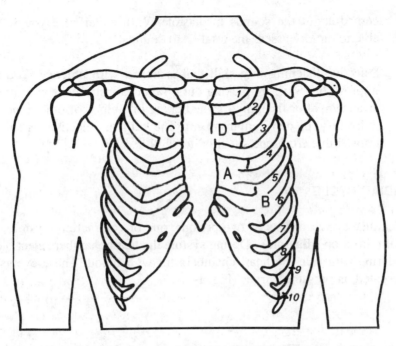

**Fig. I-3.**   Sites for auscultation: **A,** *left lateral sternal border* (sounds from tricuspid valve and right side of heart heard best); **B,** *apex* (sounds from mitral valve and left side of heart heard best); **C,** *base right* (sounds from aortic valve heard best); **D,** *base left* (sounds from pulmonic valve heard best).

     b. Apex: This is the fifth intercostal space (5 ICS) in the midclavic-ular line. Sounds from the mitral valve and left heart are heard best.

     c. Base right (previously known as aortic area): This is the second intercostal space (2 ICS) to the right of the sternum. Sounds from the aortic valve are heard best.

     d. Base left (previously known as pulmonic area): This is the second intercostal space (2 ICS) to the left of the sternum. Sounds from the pulmonic valve are heard best.

7. **Use a sequence for auscultation.** Each time you listen to a heart, begin at the same cardiac area. Listen to all of the previously men-tioned four areas, using the same order each time. This will help you establish a routine for yourself; you will "automatically" listen to all four areas each time you auscultate a heart. The order in which you listen is an individual preference. If you already have established such a personal preference, please do not feel obliged to change it.

8. **Use selective listening.** Listen to one thing at a time. When listening to the first heart sound ($S_1$), do not be concerned about the second heart sound ($S_2$). If listening to sounds in systole, do not be con-

cerned about the sounds in diastole. With experience you will be able to rapidly assess the total heart sounds.

Selective listening is a skill that is honed with practice. You may improve this skill by picking out a favorite instrument in a musical arrangement or listening for the ticking of a clock or other repetitive noise in your daily environment. The skill of selective listening is transferable from one situation to another.

## CARDIAC CYCLE

The cardiac cycle consists of two periods: one of contraction (**systole**) and one of relaxation (**diastole**). During **systole** the heart chambers eject blood, and during **diastole** the heart chambers fill with blood. These events are represented on pressure curves (Fig. 1-4).

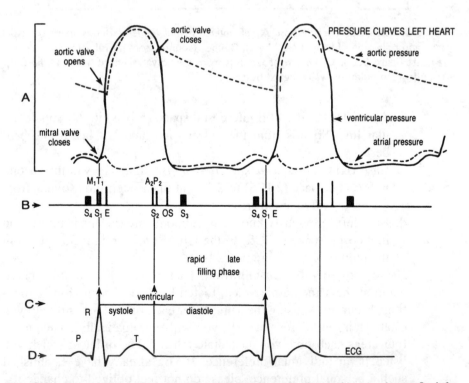

**Fig. I-4.**   Time relationships of various cardiac events. From the top down: **A,** left heart pressure curves—aortic, ventricular, and atrial; **B,** heart sounds—normal ($S_1$, $S_2$) and extra ($S_4$, ejection [E], opening snap [OS], and $S_3$); **C,** cardiac cycle—ventricular systole and diastole; **D,** electrocardiogram (ECG).

**Ventricular systole** follows closure of the mitral and tricuspid valves. This systolic period is divided into two phases:

1. The first part of the systolic period has two subdivisions.
   a. This period begins with the first initial rise in ventricular pressure after the closure of the mitral and tricuspid valves. It also is known as the **isovolumic contraction phase.**
   b. It is followed by **rapid ventricular ejection,** which occurs when ventricular pressure exceeds the pressure in the aorta and the pulmonary artery. This forces the aortic and pulmonic valves to open, causing blood to be rapidly ejected from the ventricles.
2. During the latter part of ventricular systole, ventricular pressure falls, and reduced ventricular ejection occurs. This period lasts until ventricular ejection stops and ventricular diastole begins.

**Ventricular diastole** follows closure of the aortic and pulmonic valves. This diastolic period is divided into the following three phases:

1. The first third of the diastolic period has two subdivisions.
   a. Initially in this period no blood enters the ventricles; therefore they do not increase in volume. This also is known as the **isovolumic relaxation phase.**
   b. When atrial pressure exceeds ventricular pressure, the mitral and tricuspid valves open, and blood rapidly enters the ventricles. This also is known as the **rapid filling phase.**
2. During the middle third of the diastolic period, there is almost no inflow into the ventricles. This is the period during which both the atrium and the ventricles are relaxed.
3. During the last third of the diastolic period, atrial contraction or "atrial kick" occurs, and the remaining blood is squeezed from the atrium. This also is known as the **late filling phase.**

**Atrial systole** occurs during the last third of ventricular diastole. Atrial systole may contribute 20% to 25% to ventricular filling. The contribution is less at faster heart rates (100 beats per minute or greater).

## CARDIAC SOUND-CYCLE RELATIONSHIP

Cardiac sounds are named according to their sequence of occurrence and are produced at specific points in the cardiac cycle. The initial sound heard is the **first heart sound,** or $S_1$. It occurs at the beginning of ventricular systole when ventricular volume is maximal. The sound occurring at the end of ventricular systole is the **second heart sound,** or $S_2$. The period between

$S_1$ and $S_2$ represents ventricular systole; the period following $S_2$ and the next $S_1$ represents ventricular diastole (see Fig. 1-4).

## CARDIAC VALVE AREAS

Sounds from the heart valves (mitral, tricuspid, aortic, and pulmonic) are heard at specific areas on the chest. As previously discussed:

1. Mitral valve sounds and other left heart sounds are heard best at the apex.
2. Tricuspid valve sounds and other right heart sounds are heard best at the LLSB.
3. Aortic valve sounds are heard best at base right.
4. Pulmonic valve sounds are heard best at base left.

The anatomic location of the valve and the auscultatory area (area heard best) are not synonymous (see Fig. 6-1).

The amount of energy behind the heart sound's production is a contributory factor behind its auscultatory area. Since left heart sounds have more energy behind their productions, they are audible anywhere on the precordium. Right heart sounds, with less energy behind their productions, usually are heard best only at one area—the site to which they radiate.

## CARDIAC SOUND PRODUCTION

Cardiac sound production results from at least two basic mechanisms:

1. The sudden acceleration or deceleration of blood, which is mainly influenced by:
   a. The opening and closing of heart valves
   b. Sudden tension of intracardiac structures (e.g., chordae tendineae, papillary muscles, or chamber walls)
2. Turbulent blood flow, produced when anatomically there is one of the following:
   a. Unilateral protrusion into the bloodstream
   b. Circumferential narrowing
   c. Flow into a distal chamber of larger diameter than the proximal chamber
   d. Flow into a distal chamber of smaller diameter than the proximal chamber
   e. High flow rates
   f. Abnormal communications (e.g., ventricular septal defect, atrial septal defect)

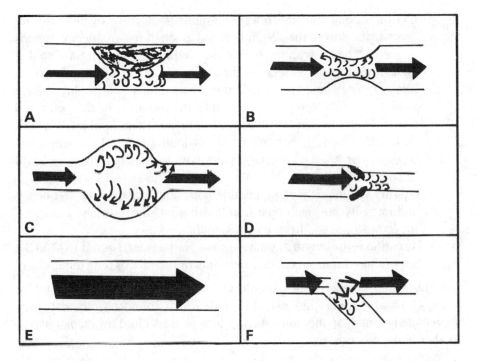

**Fig. 1-5.** Factors producing turbulence: **A,** unilateral protrusion into the bloodstream; **B,** circumferential narrowing; **C,** distal chamber larger than proximal one; **D,** distal chamber smaller than proximal one; **E,** high flow rates; **F,** abnormal communications (i.e., VSD).

These conditions can cause eddies in the vascular system and produce vibrations that are audible (Fig. 1-5).

## CHARACTERISTICS OF SOUND

Four basic characteristics of sound must be considered: (1) frequency, (2) intensity, (3) quality, and (4) duration.

1. **Frequency** is the number of wave cycles generated per second by a vibrating body. It is vibratory movement of an object in motion that initiates the sound wave cycles that can be discerned with the stethoscope. Frequency determines **pitch,** a subjective sensation that indicates to the listener whether the tone is high or low on a musical scale.
   a. High frequency—the greater the number of wave cycles per second, the higher the frequency and the pitch. High frequency sounds are best heard with the diaphragm of the stethoscope applied firmly, so that an after-imprint is seen on the chest.

     b. Low frequency—the fewer the number of wave cycles per second, the lower the frequency and pitch. Low-frequency sounds are best heard with the bell of the stethoscope held lightly so that no after-imprint is seen on the chest.

2. **Intensity** is related to the height of the sound wave produced by a vibrating object. Intensity determines the loudness of the perceived sound. High-amplitude waves are produced when an object vibrates with great energy; they are heard as loud sounds. Low-amplitude waves occur when an object vibrates with low energy; they are heard as soft sounds.

3. **Quality** distinguishes two sounds with equal degrees of frequency and intensity but that come from a different source (piano from violin or heart sounds from breath sounds).

4. **Duration** is the length of time the sound lasts. Heart sounds ($S_1$ and $S_2$) are of short duration. Cardiac murmurs or rubs are of long duration.

These four characteristics should be considered when listening to the heart. Only with experience can the subtleties of sound characteristics be appreciated—much as the quiet stirring of a restless child awakens only its mother while others sleep.

## SOUND TRANSMISSION

Three factors enter into how well a sound is transmitted from its source to the auscultator's ears: (1) the type of substance through which it travels, (2) the quality of the stethoscope, and (3) the human ear.

1. **Types of substances**
   a. Bone is an excellent transmitter of sound.
   b. Blood and muscle are fair transmitters.
   c. Air is a poor transmitter. Therefore the lung, which is normally filled with air, is a poor transmitter of sound. During cardiac auscultation, the heart sounds are heard best in individuals with thin chests because the sounds are being transmitted primarily by blood, muscle, or bone. Cardiac auscultation is more difficult in individuals with thick chests. Obesity, or increased adipose tissue, will decrease sound transmission, as will conditions that cause increased anterior-posterior (A-P) diameter from air-trapping (chronic obstructive lung disease).

2. **Quality of the stethoscope**
   The stethoscope chosen must be of good quality and have both a bell and a diaphragm chestpiece or one that combines the bell and

diaphragm modes into a single-side chestpiece. The quality of the sound transmitted is affected by the design and structural factors of the stethoscope. The tubing of the stethoscope must permit the heart sounds to be transmitted to the ears without loss of quality or the introduction of ambient noises from the environment. Whether to use a scope with a double or single tube is debatable. Theoretically sound transmission is better with the double tube, although there is some difference of opinion on this. The single-tube stethoscope has certain mechanical advantages: less bulk, less ambient noise from the tubes rubbing on each other, and a smaller surface to pick up outside noise. The length of the tubing should be as short as feasible for the clinical situation in which it is used routinely. Regardless of the type of stethoscope chosen, the earpieces must fit the examiner's ear canal comfortably; they should be neither too tight nor too loose. Very small ear tips penetrate deeply into the canals, actually causing pain; very large tips may occlude the canals. Neither fit facilitates auscultation.

Amplifying stethoscopes are available, and some clinicians may find them of value. However, in any system with amplification, the heart sounds may be different from the way they ordinarily are heard with the binaural stethoscope. This may cause difficulty in interpreting the sounds and in differentiating the artifact inherent in the instrument from true normal or abnormal heart sounds.

Regardless of the stethoscope chosen, the most important part is that between the two earpieces. A quality stethoscope in the hands of an individual prepared to use it is an invaluable instrument.

3. **The human ear**

Individuals differ in their ability to hear. The normal human ear is capable of perceiving sounds with a frequency of 20 to 20,000 cycles/second and a duration of as little as 0.02 second. The audible components of heart sounds and murmurs are in the frequency range between 30 to 250 cycles/second. Because of the peculiarities of the human ear, high-frequency sounds may seem louder than a low-frequency sound of equal intensity. Also, very loud sounds may momentarily deafen. Therefore the auscultator may have trouble hearing a soft sound that immediately follows a loud sound.

High-frequency perception decreases with age, but this should not interfere with cardiac auscultation because heart sounds are in the lower-frequency range of the hearing capability of the ear. This means that the ability to hear heart sounds should improve with age.

## CLASSIFICATION OF SOUNDS AND MURMURS

Sounds and murmurs may be classified on a one-through-six scale as follows:

1. Not audible during the first few seconds of auscultation; heard after listener tunes in
2. Heard immediately, but faint
3. Loud but without a thrust or thrill
4. Loud with a thrust or thrill
5. Loud with a thrust or thrill and audible with the chestpiece tilted on the chest
6. Loud with a thrust or thrill and audible with the chestpiece just off the chest wall

"Thrust" is an *intermittent* palpable (sometimes even visible) sensation at the site being auscultated. This is the sensation felt when palpating the point of maximal impulse at the apex of the heart. "Thrill" is a *continuous* palpable sensation comparable to the vibration felt when a cat purrs.

To chart a sound or murmur, a fraction is used ($\frac{3}{6}$ or $^{III}\!/_{VI}$). The numerator of the fraction indicates where the sound being described fits into the classification system. The denominator indicates the total number of parts in the classification. Therefore a sound described as a $\frac{3}{6}$ would be one that is loud but without a thrust or thrill (as indicated by the numerator "3"). It is being described in a classification system with six parts (as indicated by the denominator "6").

## CHARTING HEART SOUNDS

When charting heart sounds, a description of what is heard at each of the four basic auscultatory sites is given. Included in the description are the sound characteristics of frequency, intensity, quality, and duration. In addition, the charting should include:

1. Area of auscultation—LLSB, apex, base right, base left
2. Heart rate
3. Patient's position—e.g., supine, sitting, left lateral recumbent
4. Description of $S_1$ and $S_2$
5. Presence of other sounds—splits, ejection sounds, clicks, $S_3$, $S_4$
6. Presence of murmurs—noting the following:
    a. Location of valve area where murmur is heard best
    b. Loudness (intensity) by using one-through-six classification
    c. Frequency (pitch)—low, medium, high

    d. Quality—blowing, harsh or rough, or rumble

    e. Timing—systolic or diastolic

    f. Finer timing—early, mid, late, or pan

    g. Radiation—other locations murmur is heard

    h. Increase or decrease of murmur with respiration, position, special maneuvers, or drugs

7. The type of stethoscope chestpiece used—bell or diaphragm
8. The effect of respiration or other maneuvers—inspiration or expiration (e.g., standing, squatting, Valsalva)

The auscultogram, a graphic method of charting heart sounds, is one of the easiest methods to use. The auscultogram provides an easy means of drawing what is heard during cardiac auscultation. The auscultogram includes the following:

1. A drawing of the chest with the four basic auscultatory sites marked
2. Blank blocks drawn one on top of the other six blocks high; (each block represents one classification in the grading system, with one being the bottom block and six being the top block)
3. $S_1$ and $S_2$ represented by vertical lines drawn in the blank blocks to indicate the intensity of the sounds
4. $S_3$, $S_4$, splits, clicks, and ejection sounds if heard
5. Murmurs, which are represented by sine waves:

    a. Widely spaced for low frequency

    b. Close picket fence lines for high frequency

The loudness is represented by the height of the wave on a one-through-six scale (Fig. 1-6).

## MIMICKING SOUNDS

The quality of cardiac sounds can only be captured by the human ear. Phonocardiography produces visual records but not sound. Trying to appreciate heart sounds by looking at a phonocardiogram would be like trying to appreciate a symphony by merely reading the score. The sounds are transcribed, but the music is lost.

A vocabulary that translates the cardiac sounds into spoken syllables has been developed. The normal heart cycle produces a two-sound cadence that can be simulated by the syllables "lub" and "dub." The prefix "l" is used to represent $S_1$—"lub"; the prefix "d" is used to represent $S_2$—"dub." Extra sounds such as $S_3$, $S_4$, clicks, and snaps are represented by the prefix "b." The intensity of the sounds is represented as follows on p. 15:

Name _____ Date _____

## AUSCULTOGRAM

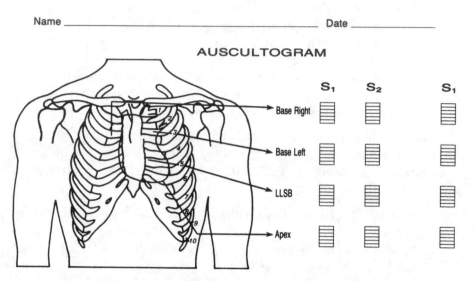

Indicate the loudness of the $S_1$ and $S_2$ at each of the auscultatory sites by drawing vertical lines to the appropriate height in the blank blocks using the one-through-six scale:

(Each block represents one classification in the grading system.
"1" being the bottom block and "6" being the top block.)

1. Not audible during the first few seconds of auscultation.
2. Heard immediately, but faint.
3. Loud but without a *thrust or thrill.
4. Loud but with a thrust or thrill.
5. Loud with a thrust or thrill and audible with the chestpiece tilted on the chest.
6. Loud with a thrust or thrill and audible with chestpiece just off the chest wall.

*"Thrill" is a *continuous* palpable sensation comparable to the vibration felt when a cat purrs; "thrust" is an intermittent palpable, sometimes even visible, sensation at the site being ascultated.

Draw in extra sound [i.e., $S_3$,$S_4$, ejection (E), or clicks (C)] as indicated.

Draw murmurs in the appropriate cycle.

Use the following sine waves to indicate the frequency/quality:

Use the one-through-six scale indicate loudness of murmur by drawing sine wave to height comparable to the loudness of the murmur.

High Frequency = ‖‖‖‖‖‖‖‖‖
(Blowing)

Low Frequency = ∿∿∿∿∿∿
(Rumbling)

Mixture = ∿‖‖‖∿‖

**Fig. 1-6.** An auscultogram, a graphic method of recording heart sounds and murmurs.

| $S_1$ | $S_2$ | Extra sounds |
|---|---|---|
| 1. Faint sounds-----------"le" | "de" | "be" |
| 2. Normal sounds--------"lub" | "dub" | "bub" |
| 3. Loud sounds-----------"lup" | "dup" | "bup" |
| 4. Very loud sounds -----"lupp" | "dupp" | "bupp" |

The cadence for a normal $S_4$ $S_1$ $S_2$ would be mimicked by syllables "bub" "lub" "dub." The cadence for a soft $S_4$ followed by a normal $S_1$ $S_2$ would be vocalized as "be" "lub" "dub"; a normal $S_1$ and $S_2$ with a loud $S_3$ would be vocalized as "lub" "dub" "bupp."

## ≡ SELF-LEARNING QUESTIONS

Select the letter of the correct response or provide requested information. Compare your answers with the answer key at the end of the chapter. Reread the chapter as needed to achieve mastery of the content.

1. Name five of the eight requirements for adequate cardiac auscultation.
   a.
   b.
   c.
   d.
   e.

2. Cardiac sounds and murmurs of low frequency can be heard best by using
   a. a diaphragm chestpiece
   b. a monaural scope
   c. a bell chestpiece
   d. either a bell or diaphragm chestpiece

3. The two basic mechanisms of cardiac sound production are
   a.
   b.

4. The number of wave cycles generated per second by a vibrating body is a description of the sound characteristic of
   a. quality
   b. intensity
   c. frequency
   d. duration

5. The best type of substance for transmitting sound is
   a. blood
   b. fat
   c. air
   d. bone

6. The frequency perception that is decreased with aging is
   a. low
   b. medium
   c. high
   d. none

7. At which area of the chest would mitral or left heart sounds be heard best?
   a. left lateral sternal border
   b. apex
   c. base right
   d. base left

8. The rapid filling phase, when the mitral and tricuspid valves open and blood rapidly enters the ventricles, is a part of
   a. atrial systole
   b. atrial diastole
   c. ventricular systole
   d. ventricular diastole

9. The cardiac sound that occurs at the beginning of ventricular systole when ventricular volume is maximal is called the
   a. first sound ($S_1$)
   b. second sound ($S_2$)
   c. third sound ($S_3$)
   d. fourth sound ($S_4$)

10. Indicate the graphic representation of a cardiac sound that is loud without a thrill by drawing lines at the appropriate height in the following box.

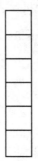

======  **ANSWERS TO SELF-LEARNING QUESTIONS**

1. Any five of the following eight responses:
   —A quiet, well-lit, warm room
   —A properly disrobed patient
   —Examine in three positions—supine, sitting, and left lateral recumbent
   —Use a stethoscope with a bell and diaphragm chestpiece
   —Listen to at least four basic areas
   —Use a sequence for auscultation
   —Use selective listening
   —Examine patient from right side

2. c

**3.** —The sudden acceleration or deceleration of blood
    —Turbulent blood flow

**4.** c

**5.** d

**6.** c

**7.** b

**8.** d

**9.** a

**10.**

# CHAPTER 2

## *The First Heart Sound (S₁)*

**LEARNING OBJECTIVES**

After reading this chapter, listening to the accompanying audio program, answering the self-learning questions at the end of the chapter, and listening to the "unknowns" on the audio program, the learner will be able to do the following:

1. Identify the classical theory behind the production of the $S_1$
2. Differentiate between a single $S_1$ and a normal split $S_1$
3. Recognize a normal $S_1$ at the various auscultatory sites
4. Identify the physiological factors that affect the intensity of $S_1$
5. Identify methods of differentiating $S_1$ from $S_2$

## COMPONENTS OF S$_1$

The *classical* and generally accepted theory for the production of S$_1$ is that S$_1$ is associated with the closure of the mitral (M$_1$) and tricuspid (T$_1$) valves. The **latest** theory indicates that it is the change in the rate of pressure rise in the ventricles, causing sudden tension of intracardiac structures, that contributes to the first heart sound production. The classical theory, although not entirely true, is "simple" and easily correlated with clinical findings and therefore will be used for the text. Since S$_1$ is caused by the closure of two separate valves, both must be considered when listening to it.

   **M$_1$** is the first audible component of S$_1$. This component normally occurs before T$_1$. (Left-sided mechanical events occur before right-sided mechanical events.) M$_1$ occurs just after the mitral valve closes. This occurs approximately 0.02 to 0.03 second after left ventricular pressure equals left atrial pressure. M$_1$ is of slightly higher intensity and frequency than T$_1$ and is discernible at all the auscultatory sites, but is heard best at the apex. Since it is a high-frequency sound, it is heard best with the diaphragm pressed firmly.

   **T$_1$** is the second component of S$_1$. It normally follows M$_1$ just after the tricuspid valve closes. Since there is less energy behind the production of this sound, it may be heard only at the left lateral sternal border (LLSB), the area to which T$_1$ radiates or is heard best. Since it is a high-frequency sound, it is heard best with the diaphragm applied firmly.

## SPLIT S$_1$

When both components that make S$_1$ (M$_1$ and T$_1$) are separately distinguishable, it is known as a **split.** In a normal split S$_1$, the components making the sound are 0.02 second apart. (Fig. 2-1)

   The separation between sounds must be at least 0.02 second or greater for the human ear to hear two definite sounds. Since the normal distance between M$_1$ and T$_1$ is *only* 0.02 second, a normally split S$_1$ may be difficult to hear. The ear may perceive it as "slurred" or "fuzzy" and not two separate sounds.

   ❖ Listen now to an S$_1$ that is split at various distances. The initial split will be 0.08 second—the ear will hear two definite sounds. Gradually the interval of the split decreases—0.06 second; then 0.04 second; then 0.02 second (the duration of the normal split S$_1$). Practice listening until

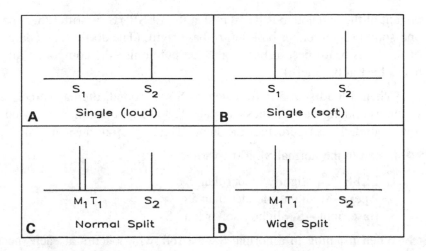

**Fig. 2-1.** Splitting of the first heart sound (S₁): **A,** single first sound (S₁) louder than the second (S₂); **B,** single S₁ softer than S₂; **C,** normal split first sound (M₁T₁) 0.02 second; **D,** wide split first sound (M₁T₁) 0.04 second. (Reproduced with permission from L. Caccamo and B. Erickson, *Cardiac auscultation,* Youngstown, Ohio: St. Elizabeth Hospital Medical Center, 1975.)

you perceive the difference between a single S₁ (only one component audible) and a split S₁ (both components audible).

In a normal heart, the split S₁ may be audible only when listening over the area to which the softer tricuspid component radiates—the LLSB. Although a split S₁ is commonly heard in children, it is heard only in about half of normal adults. To be considered a normal split S₁, M₁, and T₁ must be of high frequency and heard close together—0.02 second apart. The split is not affected markedly by respiration. When audible, it is heard consistently.

❖ Listen now to a normal S₁ at the various sites.

   1. LLSB—split or single S₁ heard
   2. Apex—single S₁ heard
   3. Base right—single S₁ heard
   4. Base left—single S₁ heard

## INTENSITY OF FIRST SOUND (S₁)

The **intensity,** or loudness, of S₁ also changes, depending on the site auscultated. S₁ always is slightly louder than S₂ at either the LLSB or the apex. (The M₁ component of the first sound is heard best at the apex; the T₁ component of the first sound is heard best at the LLSB.) $S_1$ is softer than the second sound ($S_2$) at either base left or base right. (The aortic ($A_1$) component of the $S_2$ is heard best at base right; the pulmonic ($P_1$) component of $S_2$ is heard best at base left.)

When a loud sound is followed by a soft sound, the ear perceives the sound as coming **down** a musical scale. When a soft sound is followed by a loud sound, the ear perceives the sound as going **up** a musical scale.

❖ Listen to the normal $S_1$ at the various sites:

1. LLSB—$S_1$ slightly louder than $S_2$
2. Apex—$S_1$ slightly louder than $S_2$
3. Base right—$S_1$ slightly softer than $S_2$

❖ When listening to a normal $S_1$, the following occurs at each specified site:

1. LLSB—single $S_1$ or split $S_1$ louder than $S_2$
2. Apex—single $S_1$ louder than $S_2$
3. Base right—single $S_1$ softer than $S_2$
4. Base left—single $S_1$ softer than $S_2$

The intensity of $S_1$ may be affected by the following physiological factors as well:

1. **The anatomy of the chest.** Sounds are easier to hear and therefore louder in patients with thin chests. Sounds are harder to hear and therefore softer in patients with thick chests.
2. **The vigor of ventricular contraction.** Sounds are louder when there is more energy behind their production, as occurs with a tachycardia. Sounds are softer when there is less energy behind their production, as occurs with heart muscle damage (myocardial infarction).
3. **Valve position at the onset of ventricular contraction.** If the valve leaflets are wide open when they are forced closed, as occurs with a short P-R interval (from onset of the "P" wave to onset of the "QRS" or "R" wave—normally 0.12 to 0.20 second), the resulting sound is loud. If the valve leaflets are almost shut when they are forced closed, as occurs with a long P-R interval, the resulting sound is soft.
4. **Pathological alteration of the valve structure** (stiffness of the valve). If the valve orifice is closed and fixed, a loud sound may be heard. If the valve orifice is open and fixed, a soft sound may be heard.

For a synopsis of the physiological factors that vary the intensity of $S_1$ and the resultant type of sound, see Table 2-1.

**Table 2–1.** Physiological factors that vary first heart sound (S₁) intensity

| Physiological Factors | Loud $S_1$ | Soft $S_1$ | Variable $S_1$ |
|---|---|---|---|
| 1. Anatomy of chest | Thin chest | Emphysema (barrel chest) Obesity Pericardial effusion Edema of chest wall | |
| 2. Vigor of ventricular contraction | Tachycardia: exercise emotion hyperthyroid fever Systemic hypertension | Extensive muscle damage (i.e., myocardial infarction) | |
| 3. Valve position at onset of ventricular contraction when valve mobile | Short P-R (except WPW*) when valve wide open with wide arc of closure ASD* when tricuspid wide open because of volume load | Long P-R when valve almost closed with narrow arc of closure | Mobitz I (regular sequential variability of sound) Atrial fibrillation CHB* A-V* dissociation (irregular variability of sound) |
| 4. Pathological alteration of the valve structure (STIFF) | Mitral stenosis†, which keeps orifice closed and fixed | Mitral regurgitation, which keeps valve open and fixed | |

*WPW = Wolff-Parkinson-White Syndrome; *ASD* = atrial septal defect; *CHB* = complete heart block; *A-V* = atrial-ventricular
†When the first sound is *loud* and the heart rate normal, then *think mitral stenosis.*

(Reproduced with permission from L. Caccamo and B. Erickson, *Cardiac auscultation,* Youngstown, Ohio: St. Elizabeth Hospital Medical Center, 1975.)

**DIFFERENTIATING S₁ FROM S₂**

When listening to the normal heart sounds, $S_1$ and $S_2$, it is important to be able to know which sound is the first and which is the second. The following suggestions will help in making this differentiation.

At a heart rate of 80 beats per minute or less, $S_1$ follows the longer pause. (The time between $S_1$ and $S_2$ [systole] is shorter than the time between $S_2$ and the next $S_1$ [diastole].) At a heart rate more than 80 beats per minute, the diastolic period shortens, becoming equal to systole, and other methods are needed to determine which sound is the first.

In a normal heart, $S_2$ is always loudest at the base. Therefore listen at the base and determine which of the sounds is the loudest—this is $S_2$. Then gradually move the stethoscope from the base to the LLSB, keeping in mind which sound is $S_1$. In this "inching" maneuver, the stethoscope is moved from an area where the sounds are clear to an area where they are not clear. It is a useful technique when multiple or unclear sounds confuse the listener.

Another method of differentiating $S_1$ from $S_2$, especially in an individual with a rapid heart rate, is to watch your stethoscope while auscultating. The stethoscope may move outward when placed at the point of maximal impulse (PMI), and the sound heard simultaneously with this outward thrust is $S_1$.

$S_1$ also can be timed by simultaneously feeling the carotid pulse while listening to the heart. The sound heard when the carotid is felt is $S_1$. (Peripheral pulses **cannot** be used for timing cardiac sounds because too great of a time lag occurs between ventricular systole and the palpated peripheral pulse.)

A synopsis of the methods of differentiating $S_1$ from $S_2$ is depicted in the algorithm of Fig. 2-2.

A big disadvantage of listening to heart sounds on an audio program is that the physiological factor (carotid pulse) that aids in sound differentiation is absent. Therefore it may be more difficult to discern $S_1$ from $S_2$. To make it easier for the learner to identify $S_1$, the rate of the sounds simulated will be 60 beats per minute unless otherwise indicated.

**CLINICAL CORRELATION**

After gaining confidence in your ability to identify the first heart sound ($S_1$), hone your ability by listening to as many real hearts as possible. Listen to the thin and the obese; to adults and children, if possible. Note the similar-

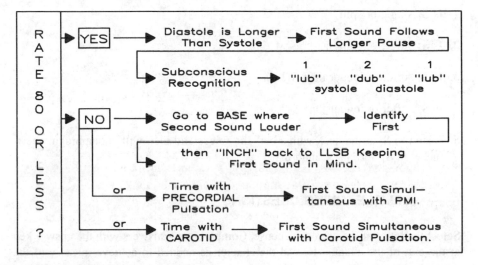

**Fig. 2-2.** Algorithm for differentiating the first heart sound (S₁) from the second heart sound (S₂). (Reproduced with permission from L. Caccamo and B. Erickson, *Cardiac auscultation*, Youngstown, Ohio: St. Elizabeth Hospital Medical Center, 1975.)

ities and differences. Attempt to distinguish a single S₁ from a split S₁. Note the difference in intensity, depending on the site auscultated. Can you differentiate S₁ from S₂ using the physiological factor (carotid pulse) available? Be selective and listen only to the S₁. The other sounds can be ignored for now. Practice recording the S₁ on an auscultogram.

In listening to patients with fever, anemia, aortic insufficiency, or mitral insufficiency, contractility of the heart is increased and the S₁ will be loud. It also is loud in mitral stenosis or when the heart expels blood against increased resistance, as in systemic hypertension. Listen carefully to S₁ in patients with these findings to see whether you can appreciate a louder-than-normal S₁.

Listen for a soft S₁ in patients with left ventricular dysfunction (myocardial infarction or congestive heart failure). Can you appreciate a soft S₁ in patients with these diagnoses?

## SELF-LEARNING "UNKNOWN" HEART SOUNDS

❖ On the audio program, listen to the "unknown" heart sounds and identify the sound. Compare your answer with the answer key at the end of the chapter. Relisten to the audio program as needed to achieve mastery of the content.

1. Is $S_1$ single or split?

2. Is $S_1$ single or split?

3. Is $S_1$ softer or louder than $S_2$?

4. Is $S_1$ softer or louder than $S_2$?

5. Listen to $S_1$ at the apex with a bell chestpiece and then with a diaphragm chest-piece. Is $S_1$ normal or abnormal?

## ≡≡≡ SELF-LEARNING QUESTIONS

Select the letter of the correct response. Compare your answers with the answer key at the end of the chapter. Reread the chapter as needed to achieve mastery of the content.

1. The $S_1$ results from
   a. opening of the mitral and tricuspid valves
   b. closing of the mitral and tricuspid valves
   c. opening of the aortic and pulmonic valves
   d. closing of the aortic and pulmonic valves

2. The intensity of $S_1$ would be greater or louder if
   a. the chest wall were enlarged
   b. less vigor were behind ventricular contraction
   c. the P-R interval were short
   d. the mitral valve orifice were open and fixed

3. In a normal split $S_1$, how far apart are the closure sounds?
   a. < 0.01 second             b. 0.02 second
   c. 0.04 second               d. >0.04 second

4. The normal split $S_1$ is best heard at
   a. base right                b. base left
   c. apex                      d. LLSB

5. To differentiate $S_1$ from $S_2$, which of the following is (are) true?
   (1) At a heart rate of 80 beats per minute or less, $S_1$ follows the longer pause.
   (2) The $S_2$ is always loudest at the base.
   (3) With the stethoscope placed on the point of maximal impulse, the sound heard simultaneously with the outward thrust is $S_1$.
   (4) The sound heard simultaneously with the palpation of the carotid pulse is $S_1$.
   a. all of the above          b. 1 and 3 only
   c. 3 and 4 only              d. 2 and 4 only

━━━ **ANSWERS TO SELF-LEARNING "UNKNOWN" HEART SOUNDS**

1. Single S$_1$

2. Split S$_1$

3. S$_1$ louder

4. S$_1$ softer

5. S$_1$ normal at apex

━━━ **ANSWERS TO SELF-LEARNING QUESTIONS**

1. b

2. c

3. b

4. d

5. a

# CHAPTER 3

## The Second Heart Sound (S₂)

The Second Heart Sound $(S_2)$

**LEARNING OBJECTIVES**

After reading this chapter, listening to the accompanying audio program, answering the self-learning questions at the end of the chapter, and listening to the "unknowns" on the audio program, the learner will be able to do the following:

1. Identify the classical theory for the production of the $S_2$
2. Differentiate between a single $S_2$ and a physiological split $S_2$ $(A_2P_2)$
3. Identify the physiology behind the normal physiological splitting of $S_2$
4. Recognize a normal $S_2$ at the various auscultatory sites
5. Differentiate between $S_1$ and $S_2$ at the various auscultatory sites

## COMPONENTS OF $S_2$

$S_1$     $S_2$

The classical and generally accepted theory for the production of the second heart sound ($S_2$) is that $S_2$ is a result of the closure of the aortic ($A_2$) and pulmonic ($P_2$) valves. Although there is experimental and clinical evidence pointing to other intracardiac factors contributing to the formation of $S_2$, the "simple" classical theory will be used in this text.

As was true of $S_1$, the left-sided mechanical event ($A_2$) has more energy behind its closure and is therefore louder than the right-sided mechanical event ($P_2$). Also, the left-sided ($A_2$) normally precedes the right-sided ($P_2$). The $A_2$ component is discernible at all the auscultatory sites, but is heard best at base right, the site to which aortic sounds radiate best. It is a high-frequency sound and therefore is heard best with the diaphragm applied firmly.

$P_2$, the second component making up $S_2$, is the softer of the two components and usually is only audible at base left, the site to which pulmonic sounds radiate best.

## PHYSIOLOGICAL SPLIT $S_2$

If both components that make up $S_2$ are separately distinguishable, this is known as a **physiological split.** The normal physiological split of $S_2$ is heard on inspiration; it becomes single on expiration. Thus respiration normally affects the splitting of the $S_2$ (Fig. 3-1). In the physiological split $S_2$, $A_2$ and $P_2$ are about 0.03 second apart. (During inspiration, there is a decrease in intrathoracic pressure that permits an increase in venous return to the right atrium. This increased blood in the right atrium prolongs right ventricular systole and delays pulmonic closing. Since $P_2$ occurs farther from $A_2$, the split becomes audible.) The respiratory variation of the physiological split is best appreciated during quiet respiration. If expiration is held, a steady state is rapidly reached until the split of $S_2$ remains fixed somewhere between the width on inspiration and expiration.

As people age, the degree of normal inspiratory splitting of $S_2$ decreases, so that many older people do not demonstrate audible inspiratory splitting of $S_2$. The absence of an audible split on inspiration does not indicate pathology, but a distinctly audible splitting of $S_2$ on expiration is abnormal.

❖ Listen now to a physiological split $S_2$—split audible on inspiration; sound single on expiration. A split $S_2$ is normal, or physiological, only if the split occurs during inspiration and becomes single during expiration. It also is normal if the split is not audible. Listen again to an $S_2$ that is split and an $S_2$ that is single (only aortic component audible).

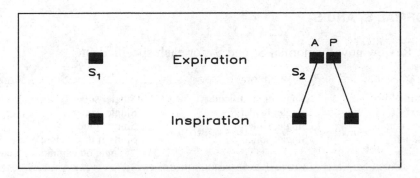

**Fig. 3-1.** Physiological splitting of the second heart sound ($S_2$). (Reproduced with permission from L. Caccamo and B. Erickson, *Cardiac auscultation,* Youngstown, Ohio: St. Elizabeth Hospital Medical Center, 1975.)

## $S_2$ AUSCULTATORY VARIATIONS

❖ Listen now to the normal $S_2$ at the various auscultatory sites:

1. LLSB—single $S_2$
2. Apex—single $S_2$
3. Base right—single $S_2$
4. Base left—split $S_2$ on inspiration; single $S_2$ on expiration

The loudness, or intensity, of $S_2$ also changes, depending on the site auscultated. $S_2$ is always loudest at base right or base left. It is softer than $S_1$ at the LLSB and the apex.

## INTENSITY OF $S_2$

❖ Listen to the loudness of the normal $S_2$ at the various auscultatory sites:

1. LLSB—$S_2$ softer than $S_1$
2. Apex—$S_2$ softer than $S_1$
3. Base right—$S_2$ louder than $S_1$
4. Base left—$S_2$ louder than $S_1$

❖ When listening to the normal $S_2$, the following occurs at each specified site:

1. LLSB—single $S_2$; $S_2$ softer than $S_1$
2. Apex—single $S_2$; $S_2$ softer than $S_1$
3. Base right—single $S_2$; $S_2$ louder than $S_1$
4. Base left—split $S_2$ on inspiration ($A_2P_2$); single $S_2$ on expiration (or always single); $S_2$ louder than $S_1$

## NORMAL S₁ AND S₂

❖ Review now the normal $S_1$ and $S_2$ for each specified site:

|  | $S_1$ | $S_2$ |
|---|---|---|
| LLSB | Single or split; louder | Single; softer |
| Apex | Single; louder | Single; softer |
| Base right | Single; softer | Single; louder |
| Base left | Single; softer | Split on inspiration; single on expiration; louder |

## CLINICAL CORRELATION

When you are confident in your ability to discern $S_2$, practice it in the clinical area. As you did with $S_1$, listen to as many different individuals as possible (e.g., young, old, thin, fat). Pay special attention to $S_2$. Can you identify whether $S_2$ is single or physiologically split? Note the difference in intensity, depending on the site auscultated. Can you differentiate $S_2$ from $S_1$? Listen selectively to $S_2$, but also listen to $S_1$. Practice recording both $S_1$ and $S_2$ on an auscultogram.

Practice hearing the normal physiological split $S_2$ that **splits on inspiration** and is **single on expiration.** You will hear it at base left. If you do not hear the split, do not think that something is wrong. The physiological split is not audible in everyone, but to be normal the split must **occur on inspiration.**

## ══ SELF-LEARNING "UNKNOWN" HEART SOUNDS

❖ On the audio program, listen to the "unknown" heart sounds and identify the sound. Compare your answer with the answer key at the end of the chapter. Relisten to the audio program as needed to achieve mastery of the content.

1. Is $S_2$ single or physiologically split?

2. Is $S_2$ single or physiologically split?

3. Is $S_1$ or $S_2$ split?

4. Is $S_1$ or $S_2$ split?

5. Listen to $S_2$ at base right with a bell chestpiece and then with a diaphragm chestpiece. Is $S_2$ normal or abnormal?

=== **SELF-LEARNING QUESTIONS**

Select the letter of the correct response. Compare your answers with the answer key at the end of the chapter. Reread the chapter as needed to achieve mastery of the content.

1. The normal S$_2$ is produced by
    a. opening of aortic and pulmonic valves
    b. closing of aortic and pulmonic valves
    c. opening of mitral and tricuspid valves
    d. closing of mitral and tricuspid valves

2. The physiological splitting of S$_2$ relates to the fact that during inspiration
    a. closure of the pulmonic valve is delayed
    b. opening of the pulmonic valve is delayed
    c. closure of the aortic valve is delayed
    d. opening of the aortic valve is delayed

3. In the normal heart, when listening at base right, S$_1$ is single; S$_2$ is
    a. split and softer than S$_1$
    b. split and louder than S$_1$
    c. single and softer than S$_1$
    d. single and louder than S$_1$

4. In the normal heart, when listening at base left, the physiological splitting of S$_2$ occurs during
    a. inspiration
    b. expiration
    c. both inspiration and expiration
    d. none of the above

5. In the normal heart, S$_2$ is louder than S$_1$ at
    a. LLSB
    b. apex
    c. base right or left
    d. base left only

=== **ANSWERS TO SELF-LEARNING "UNKNOWN" HEART SOUNDS**

1. Single S$_2$

2. Physiologically split S$_2$

3. Split S$_1$

4. Split S$_2$

5. Normal S$_2$ at base right

≡ **ANSWERS TO SELF-LEARNING QUESTIONS**

**1.** b

**2.** a

**3.** d

**4.** a

**5.** c

# CHAPTER 4

## *The Fourth Heart Sound (S$_4$)*

**LEARNING OBJECTIVES**

After reading this chapter, listening to the accompanying audio program, answering the self-learning questions at the end of the chapter, and listening to the "unknowns" on the audio program, the learner will be able to do the following:

1. Identify the characteristics of S$_4$
2. Identify the physiology behind the production of S$_4$
3. Choose the correct chestpiece of the stethoscope for listening to S$_4$
4. Differentiate right ventricular S$_4$ from left ventricular S$_4$
5. Differentiate a normal split S$_1$ from an S$_4$

## NOMENCLATURE OF S₄

The diastolic sound heard just before $S_1$ is known by the following terms: "fourth heart sound," "atrial gallop," "presystolic gallop," "$S_4$ gallop," and "$S_4$." The term "gallop" is used because at a rapid heart rate the presence of the $S_4$ in the cardiac sequence resembles the canter of a horse. "Atrial gallop" is a misleading term since the implication is that the atrium is the source of the extra sound when in fact the sound comes from the ventricle(s). $S_4$ is the most commonly used term.

## COMPONENTS OF S₄

$S_4$ is a low-frequency sound heard just before $S_1$. Since it is a sound of **low** frequency, it is heard best with the bell held lightly. $S_4$ is a result of decreased ventricular compliance or increased volume of filling. It is a sign of ventricular stress.

$S_4$ is a diastolic sound that occurs during the late diastolic filling phase (the time at which "atrial kick" occurs). Ventricles receiving this additional blood from the atrium may generate a low-frequency vibration—the $S_4$. This occurs if the ventricles have a decreased compliance or are receiving an increased diastolic volume. An $S_4$ does not occur unless atrial contraction takes place. Therefore an $S_4$ is never heard in **atrial fibrillation.**

$S_4$ normally may be heard in an athletic person younger than 20 because of the increased diastolic volume that is normal in the young. $S_4$ also may be indicative of an abnormality of the heart (myocardial infarction is associated with decreased ventricular compliance).

$S_4$ may be of either left or right ventricular origin. $S_4$ of left ventricular origin is heard best at the apex during expiration, with the patient in the supine or left lateral recumbent position. (Sounds from the left part of the heart radiate best to the apex. Having the patient supine increases the volume of blood in the ventricles, making $S_4$ louder. Turning the patient to the left lateral recumbent position brings the heart closer to the chest, also making $S_4$ louder.) Common causes of an $S_4$ of left ventricular origin are severe hypertension, aortic stenosis, primary myocardial disease, coronary artery disease, and cardiomyopathy. $S_4$ also is heard in conditions with increased cardiac output and stroke volume, such as thyrotoxicosis or anemia.

$S_4$ of right ventricular origin is heard best at the LLSB and is accentuated with inspiration. (Sounds from the right part of the heart radiate best to the LLSB. During inspiration, an increased volume of blood is returned to the right atrium and the right ventricle, making S$_4$ louder.) S$_4$ may reflect pulmonary valve obstruction, pulmonary stenosis, or pulmonic hypertension.

Dysrhythmias also may affect the presence or absence of S$_4$. S$_4$ may be heard when there is a prolonged P-R interval (0.22 second or longer) and commonly is heard in first-, second-, or third-degree A-V block. With the prolonged P-R interval, S$_4$ is not buried in the first sound or heard in conjunction with it. S$_4$ is never heard in atrial fibrillation since atrial contraction does not occur in this dysrhythmia.

S$_4$ is audible with the bell held lightly. (Pressure on the bell causes the skin to be stretched tightly across the bottom of the bell, turning it into a diaphragm.) Thus firm pressure on the bell will cause S$_4$ to diminish or to disappear.

❖ Listen now to an S$_4$. Initially only S$_1$ and S$_2$ will be heard, then S$_4$ will be added. Listen to S$_4$ with the bell held lightly, then to S$_4$ with the bell applied firmly (note that S$_4$ disappears).

**DIFFERENTIATING S$_4$ FROM SPLIT S$_1$**

S$_4$ M$_1$T$_1$    S$_2$

❖ S$_4$:
1. Low frequency before S$_1$
2. Heard best with bell held lightly
3. Pressure on bell causes S$_4$ to diminish or disappear

Split S$_1$ (M$_1$T$_1$) has the following characteristics:

1. High frequency
2. Heard best with diaphragm or bell applied firmly
3. Sounds 0.02 second apart

S$_4$ can be decreased by reducing the blood return to the atrium (by standing). S$_4$ can be increased by increasing atrial blood return (coughing, squatting, or elevating the legs) or by bringing the heart closer to the stethoscope (by rolling the patient to the left lateral recumbent position). If S$_4$ occurs from the right ventricle, it may become louder with inspiration.

❖ A split S$_1$ may be increased on standing but is not significantly affected by the other maneuvers. Again listen to an S$_4$ compared to a split S$_1$. Listen to a single S$_1$; then S$_1$ split; then an S$_4$ in front of the split S$_1$. Then listen to a split S$_1$ with an S$_4$ taken in and out.

## CLINICAL CORRELATION

Clinical practice in listening to $S_4$ can be obtained by selecting patients with conditions most likely to have an $S_4$. Patients with primary myocardial disease, coronary artery disease, cardiomyopathy, aortic stenosis, or severe hypertension may have an $S_4$ of left ventricular origin that is heard best at the apex. An $S_4$ of right ventricular origin may be heard in a patient with pulmonary valve obstruction, pulmonary stenosis, or pulmonic hypertension. This $S_4$ is heard best at the LLSB. Coronary care units are an ideal place to hear an $S_4$. (Remember that patients with atrial fibrillation can not have $S_4$.) $S_4$ changes its intensity and distance from $S_1$ during the various stages of myocardial infarction: (1) initially the $S_4$ is loud and occurs farther from $S_1$; (2) as healing occurs and ventricular compliance improves, $S_4$ becomes softer and closer to $S_1$ (therefore harder to hear); (3) if the patient has a reinfarction or an extension, $S_4$ again is loud and occurs farther from $S_1$. Therefore, in the progression of an uncomplicated myocardial infarction, you would expect $S_4$ to be initially easy to hear and to gradually become less and less perceptible. Also listen to athletic children who may have an $S_4$ that is normal. The auscultatory findings between the "normal" $S_4$ in children and the "pathological" $S_4$ are similar. The clinical history differentiates the normal $S_4$ from the pathological $S_4$. Don't be discouraged if you have difficulty in hearing an $S_4$ in the clinical area. The $S_4$ is one of the most difficult sounds to hear since it is just within the acoustical ability of the ear. To bring out $S_4$, have the patient do a mild exercise such as coughing or turning to the left side. Turning to the left lateral recumbent position also brings the heart closer to the chest wall and makes $S_4$ easier to hear. Also listen to $S_1$ and $S_2$. Practice recording $S_1$, $S_2$, and $S_4$ on an auscultogram.

### ▬▬ SELF-LEARNING "UNKNOWN" HEART SOUNDS

❖ On the audio program, listen to the "unknown" heart sounds and identify the sound. Compare your answer with the answer key at the end of the chapter. Relisten to the audio program as needed to achieve mastery of the content.

You are listening to the heart at the LLSB:
Using the bell held lightly, what do you hear?
Using the bell applied firmly, what do you hear?
Using the diaphragm, what do you hear?
1. Is $S_1$ single or split?
Is there an $S_4$?

You are listening to the heart at the LLSB:
  Using the bell held lightly, what do you hear?
  Using the bell applied firmly, what do you hear?
  Using the diaphragm, what do you hear?
2. Is the $S_1$ single or split?
  Is there an $S_4$?

You are listening to the heart at the apex:
  Using the bell held lightly, what do you hear?
  Using the bell applied firmly, what do you hear?
  Using the diaphragm, what do you hear?
3. Is $S_1$ single or split?
  Is there an $S_4$?

You are listening to the heart at the apex:
  Using the bell held lightly, what do you hear?
  Using the bell applied firmly, what do you hear?
  Using the diaphragm, what do you hear?
4. Is the $S_1$ single or split?
  Is there an $S_4$?

You are listening to the heart at the LLSB:
  Using the bell held lightly, what do you hear?
  Using the bell applied firmly, what do you hear?
  Using the diaphragm, what do you hear?
5. When listening with the bell held lightly:
  Is the $S_1$ single or split?
  Is there an $S_4$?

## ═══ SELF-LEARNING QUESTIONS

Select the letter of the correct response. Compare your answers with the answer key at the end of the chapter. Reread the chapter as needed to achieve mastery of the content.

1. The $S_4$ is of
  **a.** low frequency         **b.** high frequency
  **c.** medium frequency     **d.** rough frequency

2. $S_4$ occurs during which phase of the cardiac cycle?
  **a.** early systolic filling     **b.** late systolic filling
  **c.** early diastolic filling    **d.** late diastolic filling

3. You are listening to a patient with atrial fibrillation. You know that an $S_4$ in this
  patient is
  **a.** louder than normal      **b.** softer than normal
  **c.** always heard           **d.** never heard

**4.** Which of the following options would you choose to hear an $S_4$ best?
  **a.** bell firmly pressed      **b.** bell lightly held
  **c.** diaphragm firmly pressed      **d.** diaphragm lightly held

**5.** An $S_4$ of left ventricular origin would be heard best at
  **a.** base right      **b.** base left
  **c.** apex      **d.** LLSB

### ANSWERS TO SELF-LEARNING "UNKNOWN" HEART SOUNDS

**1.** Split $S_1$; no $S_4$

**2.** Single $S_1$; with $S_4$

**3.** Single $S_1$; no $S_4$

**4.** Single $S_1$; with $S_4$

**5.** Split $S_1$; with $S_4$

### ANSWERS TO SELF-LEARNING QUESTIONS

**1.** a

**2.** d

**3.** d

**4.** b

**5.** c

# CHAPTER 5

## The Third Heart Sound (S₃)

**LEARNING OBJECTIVES**

After reading this chapter, listening to the accompanying audio program, answering the self-learning questions at the end of the chapter, and listening to the "unknowns" on the audio program, the learner will be able to do the following:

1. Identify the characteristics of $S_3$
2. Identify the physiology behind the production of $S_3$
3. Choose the correct chestpiece of the stethoscope for listening to $S_3$
4. Differentiate a right ventricular $S_3$ from a left ventricular $S_3$
5. Differentiate a physiological split $S_2$ ($A_2P_2$) from $S_3$
6. Differentiate $S_3$ from $S_4$

## NOMENCLATURE OF S₃

The third heart sound has been known as "ventricular gallop," "protodiastolic gallop," "$S_3$ gallop," and "$S_3$." The term "gallop" was used because the sequence of heart sounds with an $S_3$ or $S_4$ resembles the canter of a horse, especially when the heart is beating rapidly.

## COMPONENTS OF S₃

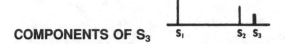

$S_3$ is a low-frequency sound heard just after the $S_2$. Because it is of low frequency, it is heard best with the bell held lightly. $S_3$ is a result of decreased ventricular compliance or increased ventricular diastolic volume. It may be a sign of ventricular distress, or trouble, as in congestive heart failure. $S_3$ is a diastolic sound that occurs during the early rapid filling phase of ventricular filling.

$S_3$ is normal in children and young adults because they have increased diastolic volumes. Men tend to lose $S_3$ in their 20s; women lose $S_3$ in their 30s. An $S_3$ after the age of 40 usually is associated with cardiac disease, except in those individuals physically active in sports. It also is heard in patients with coronary artery disease, cardiomyopathy, incompetent valves, left-to-right shunts (ventricular septal defect or patent ductus arteriosus) and is the **first clinical sign of congestive heart failure.** The preceding conditions may cause a decrease in ventricular compliance, an increase in left ventricular diastolic volume, or both.

$S_3$ may have its origin in either the right or left ventricle—the latter being more common. Left $S_3$ is heard best at the apex. (Sounds from the left side of the heart are heard best at the apex because this is the area to which they radiate.)

Right $S_3$ is heard best at the LLSB or xiphoid area. (Sounds from the right heart are heard best at the LLSB or xiphoid because this is the area to which they radiate.)

❖ Listen now to $S_3$. Initially only $S_1$ and $S_2$ will be heard, then $S_3$ will be added.

## DIFFERENTIATING S₃ FROM S₄

❖ Timing permits $S_3$ to be distinguished from $S_4$:

1. $S_3$ comes after $S_2$
2. $S_4$ comes before $S_1$

❖ In some individuals both $S_3$ and $S_4$ may be present. If the heart rate is normal (60 to 100 beats per minute) and both $S_3$ and $S_4$ are present, a **quadruple rhythm** can be heard (four-sound cadence). At a rapid rate $S_3$ and $S_4$ may occur simultaneously and are heard as a very loud diastolic sound known as a **summation gallop.** This fusion of $S_3$ and $S_4$ occurs because the tachycardia shortens diastole.

For a synopsis of the various sounds that can occur around $S_2$ and a method of differentiating one from the other, see Table 10-1.

## CLINICAL CORRELATION

Clinical practice in listening to $S_3$ can be obtained by selecting patients with conditions most likely to have an $S_3$. As was true of $S_4$, the coronary care unit is one of the best places to hear the pathological $S_3$. Remember that $S_3$ is the **first clinical sign of congestive heart failure.** $S_3$ is normal in children and young adults. The auscultatory findings between the "normal" $S_3$ and the "pathological" $S_3$ are similar. The clinical history differentiates the normal $S_3$ from the pathological $S_3$. $S_3$ is easier to hear than $S_4$, but you still may need to make $S_3$ more perceptible by having the patient do a mild exercise such as coughing or turning to the left side. Changing the patient's position from sitting to supine also may bring out $S_3$. (This also is true of $S_4$.) Having the patient grip one hand with the other also may bring out $S_3$ (or $S_4$). The hand grip increases peripheral vascular resistance, blood pressure, heart rate, and cardiac output. Also listen to $S_1$, $S_2$, and $S_4$. Can you differentiate the split $S_1$ from an $S_4$; the physiological split $S_2$ from $S_3$; $S_4$ from $S_3$? Practice recording the $S_1$, $S_2$, $S_3$, and $S_4$ on an auscultogram.

## ≡ SELF-LEARNING "UNKNOWN" HEART SOUNDS

❖ On the audio program, listen to the "unknown" heart sounds and identify the sound. Compare your answer with the answer key at the end of the chapter. Relisten to the audio program as needed to achieve mastery of the content.

You are listening to the heart at the apex:
  Using the bell held lightly, what do you hear?
  Using the bell applied firmly, what do you hear?
  Using the diaphragm, what do you hear?
1. Is $S_2$ single, split, or is there an $S_3$?

You are listening to the heart at base left:
  Using the bell held lightly, what do you hear?
  Using the bell applied firmly, what do you hear?
  Using the diaphragm, what do you hear?
2. Is $S_2$ single, split, or is there an $S_3$?

You are listening to the heart at the apex:
  Using the bell held lightly, what do you hear?
  Using the bell applied firmly, what do you hear?
  Using the diaphragm, what do you hear?
3. Is there an $S_4$ or $S_3$?

You are listening to the heart at the apex:
  Using the bell held lightly, what do you hear?
  Using the bell applied firmly, what do you hear?
  Using the diaphragm, what do you hear?
4. Is there an $S_4$ or $S_3$?

You are listening to the heart at the apex:
  Using the bell held lightly, what do you hear?
  Using the bell applied firmly, what do you hear?
  Using the diaphragm, what do you hear?
5. Is there an $S_4$ or $S_3$?

═══ **SELF-LEARNING QUESTIONS**

Select the letter of the correct response. Compare your answers with the answer key at the end of the chapter. Reread the chapter as needed to achieve mastery of the content.

1. $S_3$ is a low-frequency sound that is heard best with which chestpiece of the stethoscope?
   **a.** bell held lightly
   **c.** diaphragm held lightly
   **b.** bell applied firmly
   **d.** diaphragm applied firmly

2. $S_3$ is the result of _____ ventricular compliance or _____ ventricular diastolic volume.
   **a.** increased; increased
   **c.** increased; decreased
   **b.** decreased; increased
   **d.** decreased; decreased

3. $S_3$ is heard in an 8-year-old boy with no other abnormal clinical findings. You consider the third heart sound to be
   **a.** abnormal, needing consultation
   **c.** never normal
   **b.** abnormal, watch closely
   **d.** normal in children

**4.** S$_3$ of left ventricular origin would be best heard at
   **a.** base right
   **b.** base left
   **c.** apex
   **d.** left lateral sternal border

**5.** The first clinical sign of congestive heart failure is
   **a.** S$_4$
   **b.** wide split S$_1$
   **c.** S$_3$
   **d.** wide split S$_2$

≡≡≡ **ANSWERS TO SELF-LEARNING "UNKNOWN" HEART SOUNDS**

**1.** Single S$_2$ with S$_3$

**2.** Physiological split S$_2$

**3.** S$_4$

**4.** S$_3$

**5.** S$_4$ and S$_3$

≡≡≡ **ANSWERS TO SELF-LEARNING QUESTIONS**

**1.** a

**2.** b

**3.** d

**4.** c

**5.** c

# CHAPTER 6

## *Murmurs—General Information*

**LEARNING OBJECTIVES**

After reading this chapter, listening to the accompanying audio program, answering the self-learning questions at the end of the chapter, and listening to the "unknowns" on the audio program, the learner will be able to do the following:

1. Define a murmur
2. Identify the common causes of murmurs
3. Identify the six characteristics to be considered in murmur identification
4. Differentiate between murmurs of high, medium, and low frequency
5. Differentiate between murmurs having the quality of "blow," "harsh," "rough," or "rumble"
6. Differentiate between systolic and diastolic murmurs

## CHARACTERISTICS OF MURMURS

Murmurs are defined as sustained noises that are audible during the time periods of systole, diastole, or both.

Common causes of murmurs include backward regurgitation (a leaking valve, atrial or ventricular septal defect, or arteriovenous connection); forward flow through narrowed or deformed valves; a high rate of blood flow through normal or abnormal valves; vibration of loose structures within the heart (chordae tendineae); and continuous flow through A-V shunts.

To identify a murmur, there are six characteristics that you need to consider:

1. Location—valve area where murmur heard best
2. Loudness (intensity)—use the one-to-six grading system
3. Frequency (pitch)—i.e., low, medium, high
4. Quality—blowing, harsh, rough, or rumble
5. Timing—systolic or diastolic
6. Radiation—where else murmur heard

### Location of Murmurs

The **location of murmurs,** as with normal heart sounds, originates near a heart valve. You will find it necessary to listen to the four basic areas previously discussed, plus a fifth area, commonly called Erb's point, which is located at the third intercostal space along the LLSB (Fig. 6-1).

To determine murmur location, listen to all of the basic areas and decide at which area the murmur is heard best. You will find that murmurs from certain valves tend to be heard best "downstream" from the valve as follows:

| Valve | Heard Best |
|---|---|
| 1. Mitral | Apex |
| 2. Tricuspid | LLSB |
| 3. Pulmonic | Base left |
| 4. Aortic (systolic) | Base right |
| Aortic (diastolic) | Erb's point |

### Loudness of Murmurs

**Loudness** (intensity) is judged by using the same one-through-six classification previously discussed for heart sounds. The loudness of the murmur should not be thought to correlate with its significance. Some insignificant abnormalities may have loud murmurs; whereas the same abnormality that has progressed in significance may be softer. (Think of a plaque occluding

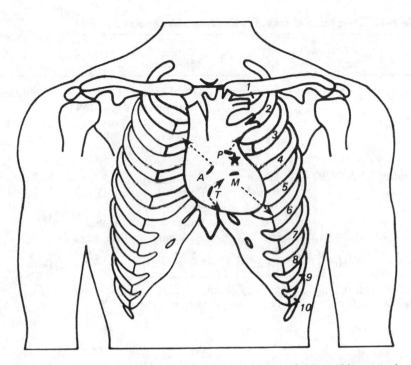

**Fig. 6-1.** Valve areas: *Anatomic* area is represented by solid bars. M = mitral valve; T = tricuspid valve; A = aortic valve; P = pulmonic valve. *Auscultatory* areas (areas where sound is heard best) are represented by arrows. Star (★) represents Erb's point.

an artery. Minimal plaque may have intense sustained noise [bruit]; complete occlusion may have no sound.)

## Frequency of Murmurs

**Frequency** (pitch) indicates whether the sound heard is high, medium, or low. This is easily determined since murmurs of high frequency are best heard with the diaphragm chestpiece; those of low frequency with the bell held lightly; and those of medium frequency with either bell or diaphragm chestpiece. With practice, the frequency of the murmur will alert you to the presence of a specific abnormality (Table 6-1).

❖ Listen now to murmurs that are considered high, medium, and low.

## Quality of Murmurs

**Quality** is closely related to frequency and is described as "blowing" (mainly high frequency); "harsh" or "rough" (medium frequency—mix of

**Table 6-1.** Differentiation of common cardiac abnormalities by pitch and quality

| Pitch | Frequency (cycles/sec) | Quality | Abnormality | Chestpiece |
|---|---|---|---|---|
| High | 200–400 | Blowing | Mitral regurgitation<br>Tricuspid regurgitation<br>Aortic regurgitation<br>Ventricular septal<br>  defect (VSD) | Diaphragm |
| Medium | 100–200 | Harsh<br>Rough | Aortic stenosis<br>Pulmonic regurgitation<br>ASD<br>Increase flow of pul-<br>  monary outflow tract | Either<br>Bell |
| Low | <100 | Rumble | Mitral stenosis | Bell |

Modified with permission from L. Caccamo and B. Erickson, *Cardiac auscultation,* (Youngstown, Ohio: St. Elizabeth Hospital Medical Center, 1975.)

high and low frequencies); and "rumble" (mainly low frequency). The quality of the murmur alerts the astute clinician to the presence of a specific abnormality (Table 6-1).

❖ Listen now to murmurs that are described as "blowing," "harsh" or "rough," and "rumble." For a differentiation of the common murmurs by frequency and quality (Table 6-1).

### Timing of Murmurs

**Timing** means that you can identify whether the sustained noise is occurring between $S_1$ and $S_2$—a systolic murmur; or between $S_2$ and $S_1$—a diastolic murmur. In some abnormalities the murmur will be heard both in systole and diastole.

❖ Listen now to a heart rate of 60 beats per minute. First, a systolic blow murmur will be added, then removed. Then a diastolic rumble murmur will be added and removed. Murmurs of different frequency and quality have been deliberately selected to help you tell the difference between systole and diastole.

As a beginning auscultator, you may not be able to pinpoint the timing any more precisely than to determine whether the murmur occurs in systole or diastole. However, with experience you'll note that even **"finer timing"** (early, mid, late, or pan) is possible. A murmur is said to be "early" if its peak intensity occurs early in the cycle; "mid" if the peak intensity occurs in the middle of the cycle; and "late" if the peak intensity occurs late in the cycle. If the murmur is heard throughout the cycle with equal intensity, it is known as a "pan" or "holo" murmur.

❖ Listen now to a heart rate of 60 beats per minute. A murmur will be added in the systolic period: early, mid, late, and pan.
❖ Listen now to a heart rate of 60 beats per minute. A murmur will be added in the diastolic period: early, mid, late, and pan.

## Radiation of Murmurs

**Radiation** of the murmur is assessed when you determine in what other areas the sound is audible in addition to where you heard it best. Each cardiac abnormality has a classical radiation. See Figs. 7-1 and 8-1 for the radiation patterns of common cardiac abnormalities.

## Shape of Murmurs

Murmurs have an identifiable **shape** to their sound that is often described in musical terminology. A "crescendo/decrescendo" (diamond-shaped) murmur starts softly, peaks in intensity, then diminishes (systolic murmur of aortic stenosis). A "decrescendo" murmur begins loud and gets progressively quieter (diastolic murmur of aortic regurgitation). A "pan" or "holo" murmur remains unchanged from the onset to the end of the sound (pansystolic murmur of severe mitral regurgitation). A "crescendo" murmur starts out soft and becomes progressively louder (late systolic murmur of mitral valve prolapse). A "decrescendo/crescendo" murmur starts out loud, gets softer, then becomes loud again (diastolic murmur of mitral stenosis).

## Special Maneuvers

**Special maneuvers** to help differentiate one murmur (or sound) from another include Valsalva, exercise, respiration, hand grip, and the use of amyl nitrate. The **Valsalva** is performed by asking the patient to bear down or strain. This maneuver increases intrathoracic pressure and decreases venous return to the right heart. Most murmurs decrease during the strain phase of the Valsalva. After release of the straining phase, right-sided events return in one to three beats, whereas left-sided events return in four to 11 beats. **Exercise** increases the heart rate and thereby increases blood flow; murmurs (and sounds) may be *increased* in intensity. **Respiration** also changes the loudness of sounds by bringing the heart closer to the chest wall and making the heart sounds louder. Therefore faint diastolic murmurs of aortic or pulmonic regurgitation may be heard better during *expiration*. [Note: This is not to be confused with the physiological effects of respiration. During inspiration, right-sided cardiac events are louder because of the increased venous return.] **Hand-grip** in which one hand is gripped with the other causes an increase in peripheral vascular resistance, blood pressure, heart rate, and cardiac output. This maneuver increases left-sided regurgitant murmurs (aortic and mitral regurgitation and ventricular septal defect) and causes left-sided ejection murmurs to decrease (aortic stenosis). **Amyl nitrate** causes a decrease in peripheral vascular resistance and increase in heart rate and in venous return. Following inhalation of amyl nitrate, *forward flow murmurs* (aortic stenosis, mitral stenosis, pulmonic stenosis, and tricuspid stenosis) *increase; left-sided regurgitant murmurs* become *softer.*

## ≡≡≡ SELF-LEARNING "UNKNOWN" HEART SOUNDS

❖ On the audio program, listen to the "unknown" heart sounds and identify the sound. Compare your answer with the answer key at the end of the chapter. Relisten to the audio program as needed to achieve mastery of the content.

Determine the frequency of the following sustained sounds:

1. This sound is heard best with the diaphragm applied firmly.

2. This sound is heard equally well with either the bell or the diaphragm.

3. This sound is heard best with the bell held lightly.
   Determine the quality of the following sounds:

4. This sound is heard best with the diaphragm applied firmly.

5. This sound is heard best with the bell held lightly.

## ≡≡≡ SELF-LEARNING QUESTIONS

Select the letter of the correct response or provide requested information. Compare your answers with the answer key at the end of the chapter. Reread the chapter as needed to achieve mastery of the content.

**1.** A sustained noise that is audible during the time period of systole, diastole, or both periods is descriptive of
    **a.** systolic murmur         **b.** diastolic murmur
    **c.** murmur               **d.** blow

**2.** Name two common causes for murmur production.
    **a.**
    **b.**

**3.** Name the six characteristics you need to consider to identify a murmur.
    **a.**
    **b.**
    **c.**
    **d.**
    **e.**
    **f.**

**4.** If the sustained noise occurs between $S_1$ and $S_2$, the murmur is called:
    **a.** systolic         **b.** diastolic
    **c.** regurgitant     **d.** ejection

## ANSWERS TO SELF-LEARNING "UNKNOWN" HEART SOUNDS

**1.** High frequency

**2.** Medium frequency

**3.** Low frequency

**4.** Blow

**5.** Rumble

## ANSWERS TO SELF-LEARNING QUESTIONS

**1.** c

**2.** Any two of the following:
    —Backward regurgitation
    —Forward flow through narrow or deformed valves
    —High rate of blood flow through normal or abnormal valves
    —Vibration of loose structures within the heart

3. —Location
   —Loudness
   —Frequency
   —Quality
   —Timing
   —Radiation

4. a

# CHAPTER 7

## Systolic Murmurs

**LEARNING OBJECTIVES**

After reading this chapter, listening to the accompanying audio program, answering the self-learning questions at the end of the chapter, and listening to the "unknowns" on the audio program, the learner will be able to do the following:

1. Define systolic murmur
2. Identify the mechanism(s) of systolic murmur production
3. Identify the characteristics of an early systolic, midsystolic, late systolic, and pansystolic murmur
4. Differentiate between an early systolic, midsystolic, late systolic, and pansystolic murmur
5. Identify common adult abnormalities having systolic murmurs

**Systolic murmurs** are sustained noises that are audible between $S_1$ and $S_2$. In some patients systolic murmurs may be normal. This may be true of babies or children because of their thin chest walls. In adults a "normal" systolic murmur may be the result of increased blood flow, as in pregnancy. A systolic murmur probably would be heard in most normal hearts if listened for in a soundproof room.

## MECHANISM(S) OF SYSTOLIC MURMUR PRODUCTION

Systolic murmurs occur during the ventricular systolic period. Forward flow across the aortic or pulmonic valve or regurgitant flow from the mitral or tricuspid valve may produce a systolic murmur. The valves may be normal (but with a high rate of flow) or abnormal. Common abnormalities in which a systolic murmur is heard include mitral insufficiency, tricuspid insufficiency, aortic stenosis, pulmonic stenosis, and interventricular septal defects.

**EARLY SYSTOLIC MURMURS**

An **early systolic murmur** begins with $S_1$ and peaks in the first third of systole. It may be caused by a modified regurgitant murmur with backward flow through an incompetent valve, a septal defect, or an A-V communication. Common causes are a small ventricular septal defect or the "innocent" murmurs of children.

❖ Listen now to a heart rate of 60 beats per minute. Then an early systolic murmur will be added.

**An innocent systolic** murmur usually is either **early** or **ejection** (see midsystolic murmurs). Its grade is a ⅖ or less. It is common in children. This sound is considered normal or "innocent" if there is no recognizable heart lesion and if the following is true:

1. Normal split $S_2$ is heard ($S_2$ splits on inspiration; single on expiration)
2. Normal jugular venous and carotid pulses are present
3. Normal precordial pulsation is present
4. Normal history, chest x-ray, and ECG exist

Common causes are:

1. Pulmonary outflow tract murmur (ejection)
2. Vibratory (humming or musical) that is heard in children (ages 2 to 7) at the LLSB

**Innocent systolic** murmurs also may be heard in the elderly, most commonly a result of sclerotic changes of the aortic valve. The murmur usually is of short duration and faint, with a grade of ⅔ or less. The "innocent" murmur of the elderly may continue a benign course for years or gradually progress and cause symptoms. Other causes of **innocent systolic murmurs** include conditions in which there is increased blood flow such as hyperthyroidism, anemia, fever, exercise, and pregnancy (92%).

❖ Listen now to a heart rate of 60 beats per minute. An early innocent murmur will be added. The early systolic murmur will be compared with a midsystolic murmur.

## MIDSYSTOLIC MURMURS

A **midsystolic murmur** begins shortly after $S_1$, peaks in midsystole, and does not quite extend to $S_2$. It is known as an "ejection" murmur. It is a "crescendo/decrescendo" murmur (diamond shaped) that builds up and decreases symmetrically. It may be caused by forward blood flow through a narrow or irregular valve such as that found in aortic or pulmonic stenosis.

❖ Listen now to a heart rate of 60 beats per minute. A midsystolic murmur will be added, which is medium in frequency and harsh in quality.

## LATE SYSTOLIC MURMURS

A **late systolic murmur** begins in the latter one half of systole, peaks in the later third of systole, and extends to $S_2$. It is a modified regurgitant murmur with a backward flow through an incompetent valve. It commonly is heard in papillary muscle disorders and in the mitral valve prolapse syndrome.

❖ Listen now to a heart rate of 60 beats per minute. A late systolic murmur will be added that is high in frequency and blowing in quality.

## PANSYSTOLIC (OR HOLOSYSTOLIC) MURMURS

A **pansystolic (or holosystolic) murmur** is heard continuously throughout systole. It begins with $S_1$ and ends with $S_2$. Since the pressure remains higher throughout systole in the ejecting chamber than in the receiving chamber, the murmur is continuous. It is commonly heard in mitral regurgitation, tricuspid regurgitation, and ventricular septal defect.

❖ Listen now to a heart rate of 60 beats per minute. A pansystolic (holosystolic) murmur will be added that is high in frequency and blowing in quality.

A review of the common adult abnormalities having systolic murmurs is provided in Fig. 7-1.

## CLINICAL CORRELATION

One of the easiest ways to gain clinical practice in listening to systolic murmurs is to seek out patients in whom these murmurs already have been identi-

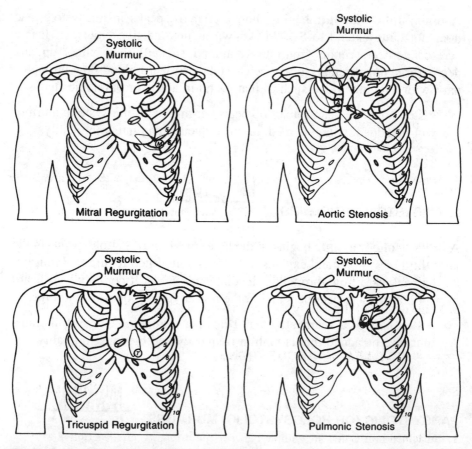

**Fig. 7-1.** Common cardiac abnormalities with systolic murmur(s): area where murmur is heard best is *circled*; area of usual radiation is *shaded*.

fied. Common pathologies having this type of murmur are mitral regurgitation, tricuspid regurgitation, aortic stenosis, or pulmonic stenosis. Patients with mitral valve prolapse may have a late systolic murmur. Systolic murmurs also may be heard in normal hearts. Initially, try to determine whether the murmur is in systole or in diastole. With practice you will be able to tell whether it is early, mid, or late in systole. Also determine the following: (1) location—valve area where heard best, (2) loudness, (3) frequency, (4) quality, and (5) radiation. Practice recording the systolic murmur on an auscultogram. Also practice writing a narrative description of the systolic murmur heard.

Keep in mind that murmurs originating on the right side of the heart generally *increase with inspiration* and that those from the left side *decrease.* You also may wish to try some of the maneuvers described in the **Special Maneuvers** section in Chapter 6.

Chapter 12, Prosthetic Valve Sounds, contains information about how a systolic ejection murmur can be heard with prosthetic valves.

## SELF-LEARNING "UNKNOWN" HEART SOUNDS

❖ On the audio program, listen to the "unknown" heart sounds and identify the sound. Compare your answers with the answer key at the end of the chapter. Relisten to the audio program as needed to achieve mastery of the content.

Listen to the following systolic murmurs.

1. Is the murmur early systolic, midsystolic, late systolic, or pansystolic in nature?

2. Is the murmur early systolic, midsystolic, late systolic, or pansystolic in nature?

3. Is the murmur early systolic, midsystolic, late systolic, or pansystolic in nature?

4. Is the murmur early systolic, midsystolic, late systolic, or pansystolic in nature?

5. Is the quality of this late systolic murmur blow or rumble?

## SELF-LEARNING QUESTIONS

Select the letter of the correct response. Compare your answers with the answer key at the end of the chapter. Reread the chapter as needed to achieve mastery of the content.

1. Sustained noises that are audible between the $S_1$ and $S_2$ are descriptive of
   a. systolic murmur
   b. diastolic murmur
   c. ejection sound
   d. friction rub

2. Regurgitant blood flow across which valves will cause a systolic murmur?
   **a.** mitral and aortic
   **b.** mitral and tricuspid
   **c.** tricuspid and pulmonic
   **d.** pulmonic and aortic

3. Forward blood flow across which abnormal valves will cause a systolic murmur?
   **a.** mitral and aortic
   **b.** mitral and tricuspid
   **c.** tricuspid and pulmonic
   **d.** pulmonic and aortic

4. Common adult abnormalities having a systolic murmur include
   **a.** mitral insufficiency and aortic insufficiency
   **b.** mitral stenosis and aortic insufficiency
   **c.** mitral insufficiency and aortic stenosis
   **d.** mitral stenosis and aortic stenosis

5. A murmur that begins shortly after $S_1$, peaks in midsystole, and does not quite extend to $S_2$ is descriptive of a(n)
   **a.** early systolic murmur
   **b.** midsystolic murmur
   **c.** late systolic murmur
   **d.** pansystolic murmur

≡≡≡ **ANSWERS TO SELF-LEARNING "UNKNOWN" HEART SOUNDS**

1. Early systolic murmur

2. Midsystolic murmur

3. Pansystolic murmur

4. Late systolic murmur

5. Blow quality

≡≡≡ **ANSWERS TO SELF-LEARNING QUESTIONS**

1. a

2. b

3. d

4. c

5. b

# CHAPTER 8
## Diastolic Murmurs

**LEARNING OBJECTIVES**

After reading this chapter, listening to the accompanying audio program, answering the self-learning questions at the end of the chapter, and listening to the "unknowns" on the audio program, the learner will be able to do the following:

1. Define a diastolic murmur
2. Identify the mechanisms of diastolic murmur production
3. Identify the characteristics of an early diastolic, middiastolic, late diastolic, and pandiastolic murmur
4. Differentiate between an early diastolic, middiastolic, late diastolic, and pandiastolic murmur
5. Identify common adult abnormalities having diastolic murmur(s)
6. Differentiate between systolic and diastolic murmurs

**Diastolic murmurs** are sustained noises that are audible between $S_2$ and the next $S_1$. Unlike systolic murmurs, diastolic murmurs should usually be considered pathological and **not** normal.

## MECHANISMS OF PRODUCTION

There are three main mechanisms of **diastolic murmur** production:

1. **Aortic or pulmonic valve incompetence.** During ventricular diastole, the pressure in the ventricles is less than that in the aorta or the pulmonary artery. If the aortic or pulmonic valves are incompetent, blood regurgitates back into the ventricles. The sustained noise of this regurgitation is the diastolic murmur.
2. **Mitral stenosis or tricuspid stenosis.** During the rapid filling phase of ventricular diastole, if the blood is forced into the ventricles through stenotic valves, a diastolic murmur occurs.
3. **Increased blood flow across mitral or tricuspid valves.** If there is an increase in volume or velocity of blood flow across the mitral or tricuspid valves during ventricular diastole, a diastolic murmur occurs.

**EARLY DIASTOLIC MURMURS**    $S_1$    $S_2$    $S_1$

An **early diastolic murmur** begins with $S_2$ and peaks in the first third of diastole. This makes $S_2$ difficult to hear, whereas $S_1$ is easily heard. It usually is a regurgitant murmur with backward flow through an incompetent valve. Common causes are aortic regurgitation and pulmonic regurgitation.

❖ Listen now to a heart rate of 60 beats per minute. An early diastolic murmur will be added that is high in frequency and blowing in quality.

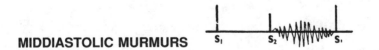

**MIDDIASTOLIC MURMURS**    $S_1$    $S_2$    $S_1$

A **middiastolic murmur** begins after $S_2$ and peaks in middiastole. (Both $S_2$ and $S_1$ are heard clearly.) Common causes are mitral stenosis and tricuspid stenosis. The murmur is low in frequency and rumbling in quality.

❖ Listen now to a heart rate of 60 beats per minute. A middiastolic murmur will be added that is low in frequency and rumbling in quality.

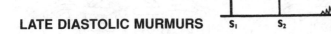

**LATE DIASTOLIC MURMURS**

A **late diastolic murmur** begins in the latter one half of diastole, peaks in the later third of diastole, and extends to $S_1$. ($S_2$ is heard clearly; $S_1$ is difficult to hear.) It also is known as a **presystolic** murmur. It is commonly a component of the murmur of mitral stenosis or tricuspid stenosis. The late diastolic murmur is low in frequency and rumbling in quality.

❖ Listen now to a heart rate of 60 beats per minute. A late diastolic murmur will be added that is low in frequency and rumbling in quality. Listen next to a heart rate of 60 beats per minute. A middiastolic and a late diastolic murmur will be added that are low in frequency and rumbling in quality.

**PANDIASTOLIC MURMURS**

A **pandiastolic murmur** begins with $S_2$ and extends throughout the diastolic period. (Both $S_2$ and $S_1$ are difficult to hear.) Patent ductus arteriosus, the prototype of aorticopulmonary connections, is a classical example of this murmur. This condition is unusual in an adult since it usually is corrected in childhood. It usually is heard best at base left and has both a systolic and diastolic component. It is therefore known as a continuous murmur. It may be heard best with the bell chestpiece.

❖ Listen next to a heart rate of 60 beats per minute. A pandiastolic murmur will be added that is low in frequency and rumbling in quality.

For a review of the common adult abnormalities having diastolic murmurs, see Fig. 8-1.

**CLINICAL CORRELATION**

To gain skill in listening to diastolic murmurs, seek out patients in whom these murmurs already have been identified. Common pathologic conditions in which this type of murmur is heard are mitral stenosis, tricuspid stenosis, aortic regurgitation, and pulmonic regurgitation. Initially, try to determine whether the murmur is in diastole or in systole. Also determine the following: (1) location, (2) loudness, (3) frequency, (4) quality, and (5) radiation.

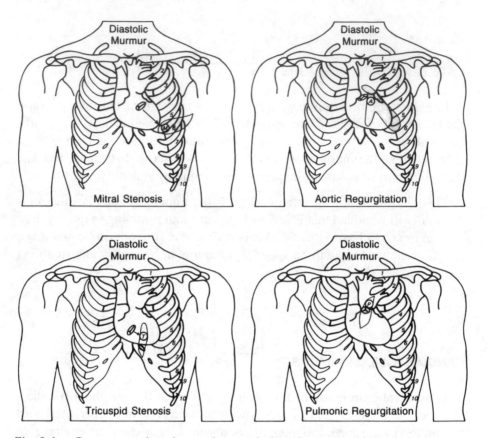

**Fig. 8-1.** Common cardiac abnormalities with diastolic murmur(s): area where murmur is heard best is *circled*; area of usual radiation is *shaded*.

Practice differentiating systolic from diastolic murmurs. Also practice recording the diastolic murmur on an auscultogram. In addition, write a narrative description of the diastolic murmur heard.

In a patient with a murmur of mitral stenosis, you may be able to hear the murmur by first finding the point of maximal impulse (PMI). Mark the PMI with a finger and then place the bell of the stethoscope lightly over this area. The typical rumble of mitral stenosis may be heard. It may be inaudible when the stethoscope is moved out of this spot. The murmur can be brought out by having the patient cough several times (a mild exercise) or simply by the exertion of the patient turning to the left lateral position. (S₃ from the left ventricle also may be heard at this identical point and by using the same maneuvers.)

Some aortic diastolic murmurs may be heard along the right sternal border (third and fourth intercostal spaces [ICS]). The development of aortic regurgitation with the murmur along the right sternal border (normally heard at Erb's point on the left sternal border) in a patient with a preexistent *diastolic* hypertension may be an indication of aortic aneurysm or dissection, or both.

### ▤ SELF-LEARNING "UNKNOWN" HEART SOUNDS

❖ On the audio program, listen to the "unknown" heart sounds and identify the sound. Compare your answers with the answer key at the end of the chapter. Relisten to the audio program as needed to achieve mastery of the content.

Listen to the following diastolic murmurs.

1. Is the murmur early diastolic, middiastolic, late diastolic, or pandiastolic in nature?

2. Is the murmur early diastolic, middiastolic, late diastolic, or pandiastolic in nature?

3. Is the murmur early diastolic, middiastolic, late diastolic, or pandiastolic in nature?

4. Is the murmur early diastolic, middiastolic, late diastolic, or pandiastolic in nature?

5. What is the quality of this middiastolic murmur?

### ▤ SELF-LEARNING QUESTIONS

Select the letter of the correct response. Compare your answers with the answer key at the end of the chapter. Reread the chapter as needed to achieve mastery of the content.

1. Sustained noises that are audible between $S_2$ and $S_1$ are
   a. systolic murmur
   b. diastolic murmur
   c. ejection sound
   d. friction rub

2. Regurgitant blood flow across which valves will cause a diastolic murmur?
   a. mitral and aortic
   b. mitral and tricuspid
   c. tricuspid and pulmonic
   d. pulmonic and aortic

3. Forward blood flow across which abnormal valves will cause a diastolic murmur?
   a. mitral and aortic
   b. mitral and tricuspid
   c. tricuspid and pulmonic
   d. pulmonic and aortic

4. Common adult abnormalities having a diastolic murmur include
   a. mitral stenosis and aortic regurgitation
   b. mitral stenosis and aortic stenosis
   c. mitral insufficiency and aortic insufficiency
   d. mitral insufficiency and aortic stenosis

5. A murmur that begins with $S_2$ and peaks in the first third of diastole is a(n)
   a. early diastolic murmur          b. middiastolic murmur
   c. late diastolic murmur           d. pandiastolic murmur

## ANSWERS TO SELF-LEARNING "UNKNOWN" HEART SOUNDS

1. Middiastolic murmur

2. Early diastolic murmur

3. Late diastolic murmur

4. Pandiastolic murmur

5. Rumble quality

## ANSWERS TO SELF-LEARNING QUESTIONS

1. b

2. d

3. b

4. a

5. a

# CHAPTER 9
## Sounds Around $S_1$

### LEARNING OBJECTIVES

After reading this chapter, listening to the accompanying audio program, answering the self-learning questions at the end of the chapter, and listening to the "unknowns" on the audio program, the learner will be able to do the following:

1. Differentiate a normal split $S_1$ ($M_1T_1$) from a wide split $S_1(M_1T_1)$
2. Differentiate a pulmonic ejection sound from an aortic ejection sound
3. Identify the characteristics of a midsystolic click
4. Identify the following:
   a. normal split $S_1$
   b. wide split $S_1$
   c. ejection sound—aortic or pulmonic
   d. midsystolic click
   e. $S_4$

**WIDE SPLIT S$_1$**    M$_1$ T$_1$    S$_2$

An abnormal split S$_1$ may result from either electrical or mechanical causes. The resulting asynchrony of the ventricles causes the mitral and tricuspid valve closure sounds to be a duration of 0.04 to 0.05 second apart compared with the normal split S$_1$ of 0.02 second. The resulting sound is known as a wide split S$_1$. The wide split S$_1$ results when the physiological split is augmented by conditions that delay pulmonic closure. Electrical causes include conduction problems such as right bundle branch block, ventricular premature beats (especially left), ventricular tachycardia, third-degree heart block with idioventricular rhythm, and, in some, pacing rhythms. The wide fixed splitting seen in complete right bundle branch block results from delayed tricuspid closure resulting from a delay in stimulation. In ventricular premature contractions and ventricular tachycardia, the asynchronous contraction of the ventricles results in the wide split S$_1$. Mechanical delays in mitral or tricuspid closure that may cause wide splitting of S$_1$ include mitral stenosis, Ebstein's anomaly, and right or left atrial myxomas. The wide split S$_1$ is heard best at the left lateral sternal border.

❖ Listen to a wide split S$_1$ as compared with a normal split S$_1$ and a single S$_1$.

**EJECTION SOUNDS**    S$_1$ E    S$_2$

Ejection sounds are high-frequency "clicking" sounds that occur very shortly after the S$_1$. They usually are heard at either base right or base left. These sounds may be of either *aortic* or *pulmonic* origin and are produced when blood is ejected from the right ventricle or left ventricle either through a stenotic valve or into a dilated chamber. Because they are high in frequency, they are heard best with a diaphragm applied firmly.

**Pulmonic ejection sounds** are heard best at base left but may be heard anywhere along the LLSB (Fig. 9-1, *A*). This sound may increase with expiration and decrease with inspiration in a patient with pulmonary stenosis. The exact reason for this respiratory variation is unknown. It may relate to pressure/volume changes between the right ventricle and pulmonary artery with respiration or be caused by the stenosed pulmonary valve opening with a "snap."

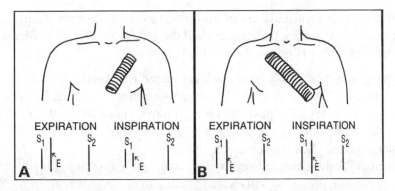

**Fig. 9-1.** Area for auscultating ejection sounds (E) and respiratory effect: **A,** *pulmonic ejection sound* (E), which decreases in intensity with inspiration and increases in intensity with expiration; **B,** *aortic ejection sound* (E), which is not affected by respiration. (Modified with permission from L. Caccamo and B. Erickson, *Cardiac auscultation.* Youngstown, Ohio: St. Elizabeth Hospital Medical Center, 1975.)

Besides being heard in pulmonic stenosis, pulmonic ejection sounds also may be heard in pulmonary hypertension, atrial septal defect, pulmonary embolism, hyperthyroidism, or in conditions causing enlargement of the pulmonary artery.

❖ Listen now to a pulmonic ejection sound compared to a single $S_1$.

**Aortic ejection sounds** are heard best at the apex but may be heard anywhere on a straight line from base right to the apex. This sound is not affected by respiration. It is heard in valvular aortic stenosis, aortic insufficiency, coarctation of the aorta, and aneurysm of the ascending aorta (Fig. 9-1, *B*).

❖ Listen now to an aortic ejection sound compared to a single $S_1$.

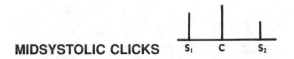

## MIDSYSTOLIC CLICKS

"Clicks" are high-frequency sounds that may be isolated or multiple sounds. Although the click usually occurs in the middle of systole, it also may occur in early or late systole. It occurs at least 0.14 second after $S_1$.

The most common cause of a midsystolic click or clicks is the ballooning of one of the mitral valve leaflets (usually the posterior one) into the left atrium at the point of maximal ventricular ejection. The click is heard when the chordae tendineae, which may be longer than normal, suddenly stop the ballooning leaflet. This is descriptive of mitral valve prolapse and is the most common cause of the midsystolic click.

Since the clicks usually are of mitral valve origin, they are heard best at the apex. They also may be heard toward the left lateral sternal border when the posterior leaflet is primarily involved.

❖ Listen now to a midsystolic click compared to a single $S_1$.
❖ Factors that reduce ventricular volume (standing, Valsalva, tachycardia, or amyl nitrite) will cause the click to move closer to $S_1$. With reduced ventricular volume, the mitral valve closes earlier after the $S_1$, and therefore the click moves closer to $S_1$.
❖ Factors that increase ventricular volume (squatting, bradycardia, propranolol, pressors) will cause the click to move farther from $S_1$. With increased ventricular volume, mitral valve closure occurs later, and the click, therefore moves farther from $S_1$ (Fig. 9-2).

For a summary of the various sounds that can occur around $S_1$ and a method of differentiating one from the other see Table 9-1.

## CLINICAL CORRELATION

The stethoscope is still the best instrument to detect and diagnose a prolapse of the mitral valve that occurs in as many as 15 million Americans. Careful listening is necessary to hear the click and the late systolic murmur (see Chapter 10) that are typically transient, intermittent, and varying. Heart disease in mitral valve prolapse is more commonly absent than present, and the majority of individuals with the syndrome are asymptomatic. Since individuals with mitral valve prolapse have increased risk of developing infective endocarditis following invasive procedures, prophylactic antibiotics are recommended before dental procedures (including cleaning, filling, and extractions), surgical procedures, and invasive procedures of the gastrointestinal and genitourinary tracts.

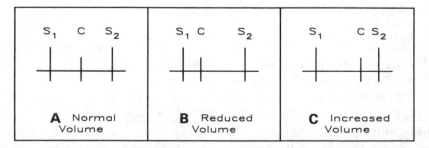

**Fig. 9-2.**   Correlation of click's distance to $S_1$ and ventricular volume: **A,** *normal* ventricular volume (click in *midsystole*); **B,** *reduced* ventricular volume (click is *closer to* $S_1$); **C,** *increased* ventricular volume (click is *farther from* $S_1$).

**Table 9-1.** Differential for sounds around the first heart sound (S₁)

| Sound Heard | Area Heard Loudest | Respiratory Variation | Chestpiece* | Change c̄ Pressure on Bell | Listen at Base R | |
|---|---|---|---|---|---|---|
| | | | | | S₁ Split? | S₂ Split? |
| Normal split | LLSB | ↑ Slight inspiration | D | None | No | Normal |
| Wide split | LLSB | ↑ Inspiration | D | None | No | Wide |
| S₄ Rt | LLSB | ↑ Inspiration | B | Decrease | No | Normal |
| S₄ Lt | Apex | → Inspiration ↑ Expiration | B | Decrease | No | Normal |
| Ejection pulmonic | Base L | → Inspiration ↑ Expiration | D | None | Yes | Wide |
| Ejection aortic | Apex | None | D | None | Yes | Wide |

*D = diaphragm chestpiece; B = bell chestpiece.

(Modified with permission from L. Caccamo and B. Erickson, *Cardiac auscultation*, Youngstown, Ohio: St. Elizabeth Hospital Medical Center, 1975.)

In the clinical setting, pay particular attention to $S_1$ and to "sounds around the first sound." Can you differentiate a normal split $S_1$ from a wide split $S_1$; from a midsystolic click; from ejection sounds—aortic or pulmonic; from $S_4$? Use Table 9-1 to help you in your differentiation.

=== **SELF-LEARNING "UNKNOWN" HEART SOUNDS**

❖ On the audio program, listen to the "unknown" heart sounds and identify the sound. Compare your answers with the answer key at the end of the chapter. Relisten to the audio program as needed to achieve mastery of the content.

You are listening to the heart at base left with the diaphragm applied firmly:

**1.** Is $S_1$ a normal split $S_1$ or a wide split $S_1$?

You are listening to a heart with the diaphragm applied firmly:
At the LLSB, what do you hear?
At the apex, what do you hear?
At base right, what do you hear?
At base left, what do you hear?

**2.** The sound you hear around $S_1$ is a:
   **a.** normal split $S_1$          **b.** wide split $S_1$
   **c.** aortic ejection sound    **d.** pulmonic ejection sound

You are listening to a heart with the diaphragm pressed firmly:
At the LLSB, what do you hear?
At the apex, what do you hear?
At base right, what do you hear?
At base left, what do you hear?

**3.** The sound you hear around $S_1$ is a(n):
   **a.** normal split $S_1$          **b.** wide split $S_1$
   **c.** aortic ejection sound    **d.** pulmonic ejection sound

You are listening to a heart with the diaphragm applied firmly:
At the LLSB, what do you hear?
At the apex, what do you hear?
At the base right, what do you hear?
At base left, what do you hear?

**4.** The sound you hear around $S_1$ is a(n):

a. normal split S$_1$                    b. wide split S$_1$
c. aortic ejection sound                 d. midsystolic click

You are listening to the heart at the apex:
  Using the bell lightly held, what do you hear?
  Using the bell firmly pressed, what do you hear?
  Using the diaphragm, what do you hear?
5. The sound you hear around S$_1$ is a(n):
   a. normal split S$_1$                 b. aortic ejection sound
   c. S$_4$                              d. midsystolic click

---

## ≡ SELF-LEARNING QUESTIONS

Select the letter of the correct response. Compare your answers with the answer key at the end of the chapter. Reread the chapter as needed to achieve mastery of the content.

1. In right bundle branch block or ventricular tachycardia, which of the following will be heard?
   a. normal split S$_1$                 b. wide split S$_1$
   c. pulmonic ejection sound            d. midsystolic click

2. A high-frequency sound that occurs very shortly after S$_1$ and is heard anywhere on a straight line from base right to the apex is descriptive of a(n)
   a. wide split S$_1$                   b. midsystolic click
   c. aortic ejection sound              d. pulmonic ejection sound

3. In a midsystolic click, factors that reduce ventricular volume will cause the click to
   a. disappear                          b. become louder
   c. move farther from S$_1$            d. move closer to S$_1$

4. A wide split S$_1$ is heard best at
   a. base right                         b. base left
   c. apex                               d. left lateral sternal border

5. A midsystolic click is heard best at
   a. base right                         b. base left
   c. apex                               d. left lateral sternal border

## ANSWERS TO SELF-LEARNING "UNKNOWN" HEART SOUNDS

**1.** Wide split $S_1$

**2.** c

**3.** d

**4.** d

**5.** c

## ANSWERS TO SELF-LEARNING QUESTIONS

**1.** b

**2.** c

**3.** d

**4.** d

**5.** c

# CHAPTER 10

## Sounds Around $S_2$

**LEARNING OBJECTIVES**

After reading this chapter, listening to the accompanying audio program, answering the self-learning questions at the end of the chapter, and listening to the "unknowns" on the audio program, the learner will be able to do the following:

1. Identify the characteristics of a paradoxical split $S_2$
2. Identify the characteristics of a wide split $S_2$
3. Identify the characteristics of a fixed split $S_2$
4. Identify the characteristics of a narrow split $S_2$
5. Identify the following:
   a. physiological split $S_2$
   b. paradoxical split $S_2$
   c. wide split $S_2$
   d. fixed split $S_2$
   e. narrow split $S_2$
   f. $S_3$
   g. opening snap

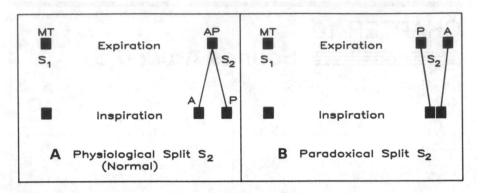

**Fig. 10-1.**   Paradoxical splitting of the second heart sound ($S_2$): **A**, physiological split $S_2$, which splits on *inspiration*, is compared to **B**, paradoxical split $S_2$, which splits on *expiration*. (Reproduced with permission from L. Caccamo and B. Erickson, *Cardiac auscultation*, Youngstown, Ohio: St. Elizabeth Hospital Medical Center, 1975.)

**PARADOXICAL SPLIT $S_2$**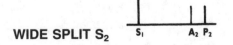

If the closure of the aortic valve is delayed, there may be a reversal of normal closure sequence of $S_2$, with pulmonic closure ($P_2$) occurring before aortic closure ($A_2$) (Fig. 10-1). Paradoxical splitting of $S_2$ is never heard in the absence of a heart abnormality.

A paradoxical split $S_2$ is identified clinically when during inspiration there is a single $S_2$ and during expiration a split $S_2$. Paradoxical, or reversed, splitting of $S_2$ may occur with marked volume or pressure loads on the left ventricle (severe aortic stenosis, severe aortic regurgitation, and large patent ductus arteriosus). With the increased volume in the left ventricle, ventricular emptying is delayed, thus delaying closure of the aortic valve. It also occurs in conduction defects that delay left ventricular depolarization (complete left bundle branch block). Conduction defects that delay left ventricular depolarization also delay left ventricular emptying, thus also delaying closure of the aortic valve.

❖ Listen now to a paradoxical split $S_2$—split audible on expiration; single on inspiration.

**WIDE SPLIT $S_2$**

The normal physiological split $S_2$ can be accentuated by conditions that cause abnormal delay in pulmonic valve closure. Five such conditions are:

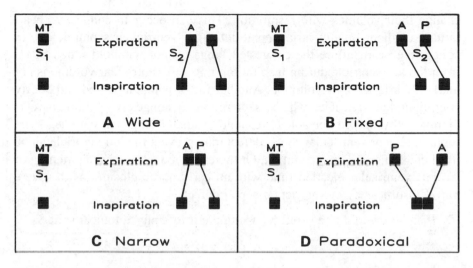

**Fig. 10-2.** Splitting of the second heart sound (S₂): **A,** wide; **B,** fixed; **C,** narrow; **D,** paradoxical. (Reproduced with permission from L. Caccamo and B. Erickson, *Cardiac auscultation,* Youngstown, Ohio: St. Elizabeth Hospital Medical Center, 1975.)

1. Increased volume in right ventricle as compared with the left (atrial septal defect, ventricular septal defect)
2. Chronic outflow tract obstruction to the right ventricle (pulmonary stenosis)
3. Acute or chronic dilation of the right ventricle caused by sudden rise in pulmonary artery pressure (pulmonary embolism)
4. Electrical delay or activation of right ventricle (complete right bundle branch block)
5. Decreased elastic recoil of pulmonary artery (idiopathic dilation of the pulmonary artery)

Early closure of the aortic valve also may contribute to a wide split S₂. Mitral insufficiency may cause early closure of the aortic valve since some of the left ventricular output is regurgitated into the atrium.

The wide split has a duration of 0.04 to 0.05 second. The physiological (normal) split is 0.03 second (Fig. 10-2, *A*).

❖ Listen now to a wide split S₂. Compare it to a normal split S₂ and a single S₂.

**FIXED SPLIT S₂**        S₁        A₂ P₂

A split that does not change its width with inspiration or expiration is called a fixed split (Fig. 10-2, *B*). It occurs when the ventricles are unable to change their volumes with respiration. This can occur in congestive heart failure, cardiomyopathy, atrial septal defect, or ventricular septal defect. In congestive heart failure the congested lungs cannot withhold much blood from the left ventricle during inspiration; thus left ventricular volume is not markedly affected by respiration. Another factor is that a dilated and poorly compliant left ventricle, which is common to congestive failure or cardiomyopathy, may not be able to respond to small changes in volume. Atrial septal defect or ventricular septal defect may prevent the left ventricle alone from changing size on respiration. Or there may be a selective shortening of the left ventricular ejection time with an early aortic closure, as in severe mitral insufficiency or ventricular septal defect.

❖ Listen now to a fixed split $S_2$. Compare it to a physiological split $S_2$.

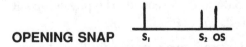

**NARROW SPLIT $S_2$**

A narrow split $S_2$ may be heard in conditions that cause increased left ventricular volume without markedly affecting the right side (uncomplicated patent ductus arteriosus with aortic regurgitation). It also may be heard in conditions causing obstruction to outflow of the left ventricle (aortic stenosis or electrical delay, as in left bundle branch block). The above conditions would cause delay in the closure of the aortic valve but would not delay closure of the pulmonic valve ($A_2$ closer to $P_2$).

With aging, the pulmonary component comes earlier, and the split narrows. This occurs because there is less blood pooling in the lungs ($A_2$ closer to $P_2$) and less venous return ($P_2$ closer to $A_2$) (Fig. 10-2, *C*).

❖ Listen to a narrow split $S_2$. Compare it to a physiological split $S_2$.

**OPENING SNAP**

Normally the opening of the mitral valve is not discernible, but under certain conditions the opening is audible and becomes known as the opening snap—a short, high-frequency click or snap that occurs after the second $S_2$. It is the result of an audible opening of the mitral valve resulting from stiffening (mitral stenosis) or increased flow (ventricular septal defect or patent ductus arteriosus). It is heard best between the apex and the LLSB with the diaphragm applied firmly. During inspiration the opening snap is softer (because of decreased blood return to the left ventricle). With increased tricuspid flow, as in atrial septal defect, a tricuspid opening snap may be heard. It is a high-frequency sound heard loudest at the LLSB with the diaphragm applied firmly. The tricuspid opening snap becomes louder with inspiration.

The opening snap is one of the early signs of mitral stenosis, and initially the opening snap is widely separated from $S_2$ (making it easy to hear). As the left atrial pressure increases, the opening of the mitral valve occurs earlier in diastole; therefore the opening snap moves closer to $S_2$. (You may then confuse it with a split $S_2$. However, the opening snap is of higher frequency and more "clicky" than $S_2$.) In severe stenosis the opening snap may merge with the components of $S_2$.

❖ Listen now to an $S_2$ followed by an opening snap.

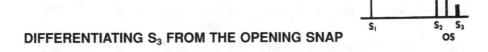

## DIFFERENTIATING $S_3$ FROM THE OPENING SNAP

❖ The opening snap occurs earlier after $S_2$ and is a **high**-frequency sound best heard with the diaphragm applied firmly. $S_3$ occurs later than the opening snap, following $S_2$ and is a **low**-frequency sound best heard with the bell held lightly. For a synopsis of the various sounds that can occur around the $S_2$ and a method of differentiating one from the other, see Table 10-1.

## CLINICAL CORRELATION

In the clinical setting, pay particular attention to $S_2$ and the "sounds around the second sound." Can you differentiate a physiological split $S_2$ from a paradoxical split $S_2$; from a wide split $S_2$; from a fixed split $S_2$; from a narrow split $S_2$; from $S_3$; from an opening snap? Use Table 10-1 to help you in your differentiation.

A technique taught by Harvey can be used to develop and sharpen your ability to detect degrees of splitting. Use your knuckles or fingers and strike two knuckles or fingers against a hard surface. By varying the degree of asynchrony, you can accurately simulate degrees of splitting from close to wide. If you use only one knuckle or finger, a single sound is simulated. (This same technique can be used to simulate $S_1$, $S_2$, $S_3$, $S_4$, or an opening snap.)

**Table 10-1.** Differential for sounds around the second heart sound ($S_2$)

| Sound Heard | Area Heard Loudest | Respiratory Variation | Chest-piece* | Change c̄ Pressure on Bell |
|---|---|---|---|---|
| Normal split | Base L | Heard on inspiration | D | No |
| Wide split | Base L | Heard on inspiration | D | No |
| Fixed split | Base L | None | D | No |
| Narrow split | Base L | Heard on inspiration | D | No |
| Paradoxical split | Base L | Heard on expiration | D | No |
| Opening snap | Apex or LLSB | ↓ Inspiration ↑ Expiration | D | No |
| $S_3$Rt | Xiphoid or LLSB | ↑ Inspiration | B | Yes |
| $S_3$Lt | Apex | ↓ Inspiration ↑ Expiration | B | Yes |

*D = diaphragm chestpiece; B = bell chestpiece.

(Modified with permission from L. Caccamo and B. Erickson, *Cardiac auscultation,* Youngstown, Ohio: St. Elizabeth Hospital Medical Center, 1975.)

## ═══ SELF-LEARNING "UNKNOWN" HEART SOUNDS

❖ On the audio program, listen to the "unknown" heart sounds and identify the sound. Compare your answers with the answer key at the end of the chapter. Relisten to the audio program as needed to achieve mastery of the content.

You are listening to the heart at base left with the diaphragm applied firmly:

**1.** Is the $S_2$ splitting physiologically or paradoxically?

**2.** Is the $S_2$ splitting physiologically or paradoxically?

**3.** Is $S_2$ a wide or narrow split?

You are listening to the heart at the apex:
  Using the bell held lightly, what do you hear?
  Using the bell applied firmly, what do you hear?
  Using the diaphragm applied firmly, what do you hear?
4. Is there an $S_3$ or a wide split $S_2$?

You are listening to the heart at the apex:
  Using the bell held lightly, what do you hear?
  Using the bell applied firmly, what do you hear?
  Using the diaphragm applied firmly, what do you hear?
5. Is there an $S_3$ or an opening snap?

## SELF-LEARNING QUESTIONS

Select the letter of the correct response. Compare your answers with the answer key at the end of the chapter. Reread the chapter as needed to achieve mastery of the content.

1. The reversal of the normal closure sequence of $S_2$ with the pulmonic closure ($P_2$) occurring before aortic closure ($A_2$) is descriptive of a
   a. physiological split $S_2$          b. paradoxical split $S_2$
   c. wide split $S_2$                d. narrow split $S_2$

2. Abnormal delay in pulmonic valve closure ($P_2$) is descriptive of a
   a. physiological split $S_2$          b. paradoxical split $S_2$
   c. wide split $S_2$                d. narrow split $S_2$

3. A split of $S_2$ that does not change its width with inspiration or expiration is descriptive of a
   a. physiological split $S_2$          b. paradoxical split $S_2$
   c. fixed split $S_2$               d. narrow split $S_2$

4. A split of $S_2$ in which the pulmonic component ($P_2$) comes earlier than normal is descriptive of a
   a. physiological split $S_2$          b. paradoxical split $S_2$
   c. fixed split $S_2$               d. narrow split $S_2$

5. A short, high-frequency sound that occurs after $S_2$ and is the result of the audible opening of the mitral valve as a result of stiffness is descriptive of a(n)
   a. physiological split $S_2$          b. paradoxical split $S_2$
   c. fixed split $S_2$               d. opening snap after $S_2$

## ANSWERS TO SELF-LEARNING "UNKNOWN" HEART SOUNDS

1. Physiologically split $S_2$

2. Paradoxically split $S_2$

3. Wide split $S_2$

4. $S_3$

5. Opening snap

## ANSWERS TO SELF-LEARNING QUESTIONS

1. b

2. c

3. c

4. b

5. d

# CHAPTER 11

## Friction Rubs—
## Pericardial and Pleural

### LEARNING OBJECTIVES

After reading this chapter, listening to the accompanying audio program, answering the self-learning questions at the end of the chapter, and listening to the "unknowns" on the audio program, the learner will be able to do the following:

1. Identify the common causes of a pericardial friction rub
2. Identify the auscultatory signs of a pericardial friction rub
3. Identify the sound characteristics of a pericardial friction rub
4. Identify the common causes of a pleural friction rub
5. Identify the auscultatory signs of a pleural friction rub
6. Identify the sound characteristics of a pleural friction rub
7. Differentiate a pericardial friction rub from a pleural friction rub

To differentiate between pericardial and pleural friction rubs, the listener must consider the following factors.

## PERICARDIAL FRICTION RUBS

### Causes

A pericardial friction rub is a sign of pericardial inflammation. Some common etiological factors include the following:

1. **Infective pericarditis.** Many organisms may cause infective pericarditis. Common ones include viral, pyogenic, tubercular, and mycotic.
2. **Noninfective pericarditis.** Myocardial infarction, uremia, neoplasms, myxedema, open heart surgery, and trauma are some of the noninfective causes of a pericardial friction rub.
3. **Autoimmune problems.** Rheumatic fever, collagen vascular disease, drug-induced (i.e., procainamide) injury, and postmyocardial injury (Dressler's syndrome) are autoimmune causes of pericardial friction rub.

### Auscultatory Signs

The auscultatory signs of a pericardial friction rub are one **systolic sound** and **two diastolic sounds.** The **systolic** sound (between $S_1$ and $S_2$) may occur anywhere in systole. The two **diastolic** sounds occur at the times the ventricles are stretched in diastole:

1. In early diastole near the end of the early diastolic filling. (This is the same time that an $S_3$ would occur.)
2. At end diastole, when atrial contraction produces sudden ventricular expansion. (This is the same time that an $S_4$ would occur.) If atrial contraction does not occur, as in atrial fibrillation, the second diastolic sound is *not* heard.

### Sound Characteristics

1. The pericardial friction rub has a scratching, grating, or squeaking to-and-fro leathery quality.
2. This rub is *high* in frequency and therefore heard best with the *diaphragm* chestpiece applied firmly.

3. The pericardial friction rub tends to be louder during **inspiration.** This may be a result of the following:
   a. The downward pull of the diaphragm on the pericardium during inspiration, which causes the pericardium to be drawn more tautly over the heart during inspiration
   b. The expanded lung pressing on the pericardium
   c. The fact that the pericardium is stretched more during inspiration than during expiration because the expansion of the right ventricle is greater during inspiration than that of the left ventricle during expiration.
4. The pericardial friction rub may be most audible in some patients during **forced expiration** with the patient leaning forward or on hands and knees. (These maneuvers cause less air to be between the pericardium and the stethoscope and also bring the heart closer to the chest wall.)
5. The pericardial friction rub is likely to be transitory or inconstant. This means that it comes and goes suddenly.
6. The pericardial friction rub may be heard anywhere on the pericardium but it is often loudest at the LLSB.
7. Most patients with a pericardial friction rub also have a tachycardia.

❖ Listen to a pericardial friction rub with a heart rate of 60 beats per minute with both systolic and diastolic sounds.
❖ Listen to a heart rate of 60 beats per minute, then only the systolic component of the rub will be added.
❖ Listen to a heart rate of 60 beats per minute, then only the diastolic components of the rub will be added.
❖ Now listen to a pericardial friction rub at a heart rate of 120 beats per minute.
❖ Listen to a real heart with a pericardial friction rub; all three components are present.

## PLEURAL FRICTION RUBS

### Causes

A pleural friction rub is a sign of pleural inflammation and indicates that the visceral and parietal surfaces of the pleura are rubbing together. Some common etiological factors of pleural friction rubs are:

1. Pneumonia
2. Viral infections
3. Tuberculosis
4. Pulmonary embolism

## Auscultatory Signs

The auscultatory signs of a pleural friction rub are **one sound during inspiration** and **one sound during expiration** (this may not always be heard).

## Sound Characteristics

1. The pleural friction rub has a grating or creaking sound similar to that heard in the pericardial friction rub.
2. This rub is *high* in frequency and therefore is best heard with the *diaphragm* chestpiece applied firmly.
3. The pleural friction rub is heard during inspiration and sometimes during expiration.
4. The pleural friction rub commonly is heard in the lower anterolateral chest wall (the area of greatest thoracic mobility) on the side of the pleural inflammation.
5. The pleural friction rub decreases with a decrease in lung movement. The sound disappears if the breath is held.
6. The pleural friction rub has a superficial character. It sounds closer to the surface than does a pericardial friction rub.

❖ Listen to a pleural friction rub in a real individual. Note the inspiratory and expiratory components.
❖ Compare the pleural friction rub to a pericardial friction rub. First a pleural friction rub, then a pericardial friction rub.

## CLINICAL CORRELATION

In the clinical setting seek out patients with pericardial and pleural friction rubs. Use Table 11-1 to help you in your differentiation. Compare the sounds of the friction rubs with those of systolic and diastolic murmurs. Practice charting your findings. If you have difficulty in differentiating pericardial friction rubs from pleural friction rubs, ask the patient to stop breathing. (It is a good idea to hold your own breath at the same time so that you remember to permit the patient to again breathe.) If during respiratory cessation the sound goes away, it is a pleural rub; if the sound remains, it is a pericardial rub.

**Table 11-1.** Summary For Differentiating Pericardial from Pleural Friction Rubs

| | *Pericardial* | *Pleural* |
|---|---|---|
| Frequency | High | High |
| Quality | Scratching, grating, squeaking | Grating or creaking |
| Chestpiece best heard with | Diaphragm | Diaphragm |
| Timing | One systolic sound; two diastolic sounds | One sound on inspiration; one sound on expiration (this may be absent) |
| | Transitory | Transitory (but less abrupt) |
| Site | Over pericardium (left chest) | Over anterolateral chest—right or left side |
| Respiratory variant | Louder during inspiration | Decreases with decrease in breathing; gone when breath held |
| Surface proximity | Farther from surface | Superficial; closer to surface |

===== **SELF-LEARNING "UNKNOWN" HEART SOUNDS**

❖ On the audio program, listen to the "unknown" heart sounds and identify the sound. Compare your answers with the answer key at the end of the chapter. Relisten to the audio program as needed to achieve mastery of the content.

You are listening at the LLSB. You hear the following sound.
1. You identify the sound as a
   **a.** pericardial friction rub
   **b.** pleural friction rub
   **c.** systolic murmur
   **d.** diastolic murmur

You are listening at the apex. You hear the following sound.
2. You identify the sound as a
   **a.** pericardial friction rub
   **b.** pleural friction rub
   **c.** systolic murmur
   **d.** diastolic murmur

## ══ SELF-LEARNING QUESTIONS

Select the letter of the correct response or provide requested information. Compare your answers with the answer key at the end of the chapter. Reread the chapter as needed to achieve mastery of the content.

**1.** Identify two of the common etiological factors of a pericardial friction rub.
  **a.**
  **b.**

**2.** One of the diastolic sounds of the pericardial friction rub occurs in early diastole; the other occurs at
  **a.** middiastole
  **c.** rapid diastolic filling
  **b.** late diastole
  **d.** none of the above

**3.** Identify two of the common etiological factors of a pleural friction rub in early diastole.
  **a.**
  **b.**

**4.** Which characteristic is most helpful in differentiating a pericardial from a pleural friction rub?
  **a.** quality
  **c.** breath-holding
  **b.** frequency
  **d.** site

## ══ ANSWERS TO SELF-LEARNING "UNKNOWN" HEART SOUNDS

**1.** a

**2.** b

## ══ ANSWERS TO SELF-LEARNING QUESTIONS

**1.** Any two of the following:
  —Infective (e.g., viral, tuberculosis)
  —Noninfective (e.g., myocardial infarction)
  —Autoimmune (rheumatic fever)

**2.** b

**3.** Any two of the following:
  —Pneumonia
  —Viral infections
  —Tuberculosis
  —Pulmonary embolism

**4.** c

# CHAPTER 12

## *Prosthetic Valve Sounds*

**LEARNING OBJECTIVES**

After reading this chapter, listening to the accompanying audio program, answering the self-learning questions at the end of the chapter, and listening to the "unknowns" on the audio program, the learner will be able to do the following:

1. Name two categories of prosthetic heart valves
2. Identify the types of prosthetic heart valves with fewer thromboembolic complications
3. Identify the heart sounds made by a caged-ball valve placed in the mitral or aortic position
4. Identify the heart sounds made by a tilting-disk valve placed in the mitral or aortic position
5. Identify the heart sounds made by a bileaflet valve placed in the mitral or aortic position
6. Identify the heart sounds made by a porcine or bovine pericardial valve placed in the mitral or aortic position

## PROSTHETIC HEART VALVES

Two categories of prosthetic heart valves, either mechanical or biological, exist today.

Mechanical heart valves have been used in humans since the early 1960s. These valves are made from a combination of metal alloys, pyrolyte carbon, and Dacron. Although their construction makes them very durable, it also makes them very vulnerable to thromboembolism. Patients with mechanical valves require anticoagulation. Because mechanical valves are more durable, they may be selected for use in young people who have a longer life expectancy.

Biological heart valves tend to be the less durable of the two varieties but have less thromboembolic complications, and therefore offer freedom from anticoagulation. Because of the valves' decreased longevity, they may be chosen for use in patients older than 65 who have a shorter life expectancy. They also are the valve of choice for patients in whom anticoagulation is contraindicated or for patients who are known to be noncompliant with drug therapy.

The sounds generated by prosthetic valves are dependent on the type of valve used, the area in which the prosthesis is placed, and whether the valve is functioning normally or abnormally. Each type has advantages and disadvantages and each has distinctive sounds and murmurs. A review of valve types follows.

After reading this chapter, consider how a prosthetic valve would change the first and second heart sounds.

## MECHANICAL PROSTHETIC VALVES

There are three commonly used types of mechanical valves that are placed in the mitral or aortic position. These are the caged-ball, tilting-disk, and bileaflet (Fig. 12-1).

### Caged-Ball

As the name implies, the **caged-ball valve** consists of a ball that moves freely within a three- or four-sided metallic cage mounted on a circular sewing ring. Blood flows through the cage and around the ball/poppet. Changes in chamber pressure cause the ball to move back and forth in its cage, opening and closing the valve. This type of valve has been in use for more than 40 years. It was the first durable mechanical valve and has an excellent record for being implanted for up to 20 years. The Starr-Edwards

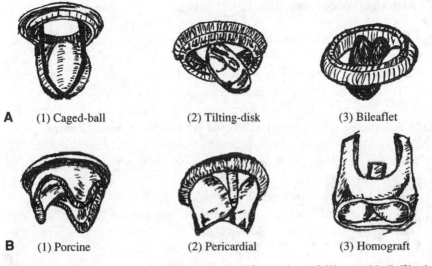

| **A** | (1) Caged-ball | (2) Tilting-disk | (3) Bileaflet |
| **B** | (1) Porcine | (2) Pericardial | (3) Homograft |

**Fig. 12-1.** Common prosthetic heart valves: **A,** *Mechanical* (1) caged-ball (2) tilting-disk (3) bileaflet **B,** *Biological* (1) porcine (2) pericardial (3) homograft

is the prototype of the caged-ball valve and is the most commonly used of its type in the United States today. Other types of the caged-ball valve include the Smeloff-Cutter, the Magnovern-Cromie, and the DeBakey-Surgitool. The Smeloff-Cutter uses a double-cage design with three titanium struts on each of the inflow and outflow regions to contain the Silastic ball. The cages are open at the apex. The Magnovern-Cromie valve is equipped with two rows of interlocking pins that are extended into the annulus. The DeBakey-Surgitool uses a pyrolyte carbon poppet intended to limit ball variance, which is a mechanical dysfunction of the prosthesis caused by physical and chemical changes in the Silastic poppets.

Caged-ball valves have a distinct, high-frequency, audible opening and closing sound that generally is described as "crisp" and "clicking" and may be audible at the bedside without the aid of a stethoscope. In the mitral or tricuspid position, there is a prominent opening "click" that corresponds in timing to an opening snap. The closing sound coincides with the first heart sound. These sounds are best heard at the apex in the mitral position; at the LLSB in the tricuspid position. In the aortic position, there is a prominent opening "click," which commonly obscures the first heart sound. When this valve is placed in either the mitral or aortic position, an early "decrescendo" or systolic ejection murmur, grade 2, or ⅜, may be heard. The murmur is accentuated in conditions that augment the stroke volume. The presence of a diastolic murmur is considered abnormal.

❖ Listen now to a patient with a Starr-Edwards caged-ball valve.

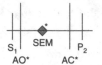

Aortic sounds:

*SEM* = Systolic ejection murmur; *AO* = aortic opening; *AC* = aortic closing.

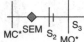

Mitral sounds:

*MC* = Mitral closing; *MO* = mitral opening.

## Tilting-Disk

The **tilting-disk valve** is a free-floating, lens-shaped disk mounted on a circular sewing ring. Depending on the type, the disk tilts open anywhere from 60 degrees (Björk-Shiley valve) to 80 degrees (Lillehei-Kaster valve) to allow blood to flow through. The tilting-disk valve allows some amount of central flow and has a low profile that permits its use in the mitral position without compromising the left ventricular outflow tract. It does not have an audible opening sound in either the mitral or aortic position but does produce distinct closing sounds. Absence of these closing sounds is abnormal. An early systolic to midsystolic ejection murmur, grade ⅔, is common. When placed in the aortic position, the sounds are heard best at base right. When used in the mitral position, the sounds are heard best at the apex.

Aortic sounds:

*┊┊┊ = Sound not audible.

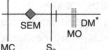

Mitral sounds:

*DM* = Diastolic murmur.

## Bileaflet

The **bileaflet valve** is the newest of the commonly used valves including the St. Jude Medical valve. It has two semicircular leaflets mounted on a circular sewing ring that open in the center. The leaflets open at an angle of 85 degrees and close at an angle of 35 degrees. Blood flow is central, and since it has a low profile it may be used in the mitral position. The bileaflet valve does not have an audible opening sound in either the mitral or aortic position but does produce a distinct closing sound. Absence of the closing sound is abnormal. A midsystolic ejection murmur is normal. In the aortic position the sounds are best heard at base right. When placed in the mitral position the sounds are best heard at the apex. In the mitral position a diastolic murmur similar to that found in mitral stenosis may be heard. The diastolic murmur is only considered abnormal if it changes or if a new diastolic murmur occurs.

Aortic sounds: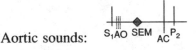

Mitral sounds: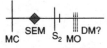

## BIOLOGICAL PROSTHETIC VALVES

Biological valves may be classified as "allograft" (isograft) from the fascia lata of the pulmonic valve; "homologous" (allograft) from an aortic valve obtained from a corpse, or dura mater; and "heterologous" (xenograft) from the bovine aortic valve, porcine aortic valve, or bovine pericardium (see Fig. 12-1). The heterologous (xenograft) currently is the most extensively used of the biological valves.

## Porcine Heterograft

The **porcine heterograft** is a porcine valve mounted on a semiflexible stent and preserved with glutaraldehyde. Blood flows almost unobstructed through a central opening. Common types are the Hancock and the Carpentier-Edwards.

### Bovine Pericardial Heterograft

The **bovine pericardial heterograft** is made from bovine pericardium fashioned into three identical cusps that are mounted on a cloth-covered frame (Ionescu-Shiley valve). Blood flow is unobstructed.

When used in the mitral position, porcine heterograph and bovine pericardial heterograph valves have crisp high-pitched opening and closing sounds. These sounds are heard best at the apex and may be accompanied by systolic murmur or diastolic rumble. When implanted in the aortic position, opening sounds generally are not heard, but closing sounds may be audible. A midsystolic murmur may be audible at the left lateral sternal border. A diastolic murmur would be considered abnormal.

❖ Listen now to a patient with a porcine heart valve in the aortic position.

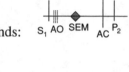

Aortic sounds:    S₁ AO SEM   AC P₂

Mitral sounds:    MC SEM  S₂ MO  DM

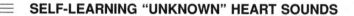

### ▤ SELF-LEARNING "UNKNOWN" HEART SOUNDS

❖ On the audio program, listen to the "unknown" heart sounds and identify the sound. Compare your answers with the answer key at the end of the chapter. Relisten to the audio program as needed to achieve mastery of the content.

**1.** Is the sound made by a mechanical or biological valve?

**2.** Is the sound made by a mechanical or biological valve?

### ▤ SELF-LEARNING QUESTIONS

Select the letter of the correct response or provide requested information. Compare your answers with the answer key at the end of the chapter. Reread the chapter as needed to achieve mastery of the content.

1. Name the two categories of prosthetic heart valves.
   a.
   b.

2. The prosthetic heart valves with less thromboembolic complications are:
   a. Starr-Edwards and Björk-Shiley
   b. Starr-Edwards and bileaflet
   c. porcine and bovine pericardium
   d. porcine and Lillehei-Kaster

3. The sounds made by a caged-ball valve placed in the mitral position include a systolic ejection murmur and:
   a. mitral opening and closing sounds
   b. mitral closing, with silent mitral opening
   c. mitral opening, with silent mitral closing
   d. silent mitral opening and closing sounds

4. The sounds made by a tilting-disk valve placed in the aortic position include a systolic ejection murmur and:
   a. aortic opening and closing sounds
   b. aortic closing, with silent aortic opening
   c. aortic opening, with silent aortic closing
   d. silent aortic opening and closing sounds

5. The sounds made by a bileaflet valve placed in the aortic position include a systolic ejection murmur and:
   a. aortic opening and closing sounds
   b. aortic closing, with silent aortic opening
   c. aortic opening, with silent aortic closing
   d. silent aortic opening and audible closing sounds

6. The sounds made by a porcine valve placed in the mitral position include a systolic ejection murmur and:
   a. mitral opening and closing sounds
   b. silent mitral opening and closing sounds
   c. mitral opening
   d. mitral closing

## ANSWERS TO SELF-LEARNING "UNKNOWN" HEART SOUNDS

1. Sound from mechanical valve

2. Sound from biological valve

≡ **ANSWERS TO SELF-LEARNING QUESTIONS**

**1.** a. mechanical
   b. biological

**2.** c

**3.** a

**4.** b

**5.** b

**6.** a

# CHAPTER 13

## Sounds After Heart Surgery and Other Sounds

### LEARNING OBJECTIVES

After reading this chapter, listening to the accompanying audio program, answering the self-learning questions at the end of the chapter, and listening to the "unknowns" on the audio program, the learner will be able to do the following:

1. Identify changes in normal heart sounds in a patient with an endocardial pacemaker
2. Identify the cause of the pericardial knock
3. Differentiate a sternal click from a midsystolic click
4. Recognize the auscultatory findings of subcutaneous emphysema
5. Recognize the auscultatory findings of an intraaortic balloon pump
6. Recognize the auscultatory findings of intracardiac myxomas

## INTRAAORTIC BALLOON PUMP

The **intraaortic balloon pump** is another commonly used prosthetic device. This counterpulsation device usually is placed through the femoral artery and is synchronized with the cardiac cycle so that it expands in diastole, displacing its volume of blood, and collapses in systole, augmenting the cardiac output. A prominent "squishing" sound is heard in systole and diastole when an intraaortic balloon pump is used and may obscure normal heart sounds.

## PERICARDIAL FRICTION RUB

A **pericardial friction rub** commonly is heard after coronary artery bypass graft (CABG) or cardiac valve surgery. This sound is loudest immediately after surgery and persists for several days and sometimes for 1 week.

A pericardial friction rub may recur weeks or months after surgery in patients experiencing postpericardiotomy syndrome. This syndrome mimics Dressler's syndrome, a postmyocardial infarction syndrome, and is believed to be an autoimmune reaction.

❖ Listen now to a patient with a pericardial friction rub. Refer to Chapter 11 for additional information on the pericardial friction rub.

The learner is advised to listen to cardiac surgery patients for pericardial friction rubs.

## PACEMAKER SOUNDS

An endocardial pacemaker in the right ventricle gives an electrocardiogram (ECG) pattern of left bundle branch block. Therefore paradoxical splitting of the second heart sound ($S_2$) may be heard. This means that $S_2$ splits on expiration and becomes single on inspiration. This splitting is heard best at base left.

If the pacing wire should penetrate the myocardium, a pericardial friction rub may be heard. Occasionally a "clicking" sound just before the first heart sound also is heard in this situation because of stimulation of the intercostal or diaphragmatic muscle. The situation can be corrected by simply withdrawing the wire into the right ventricle.

A systolic murmur may be heard if tricuspid valve function is interrupted by the endocardial pacemaker when it is going through the valve. This murmur is heard best along the left lateral sternal border and is similar to that of tricuspid regurgitation.

❖ Listen now to a paradoxical splitting of S$_2$ in a patient with an endocardial pacemaker in the right ventricle.

**PERICARDIAL KNOCK**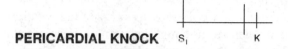

**Pericardial knock,** a sound occurring early in diastole after the second heart sound, is frequently heard in patients with constrictive pericarditis. This sound occurs slightly later than the opening snap of mitral stenosis but earlier than the third heart sound. This "knock" is a filling sound, with the pericardium acting as a constrictive membrane, preventing the usual relaxation of the ventricle in diastole.

Try to differentiate an opening snap from a "pericardial knock" or a left atrial myxoma "tumor plop."

❖ Listen now to a patient with a pericardial knock.

**INTRACARDIAC MYXOMAS**    S$_1$           T

A myxoma in the left atrium may mimic the heart sounds of mitral stenosis, except the louder-than-normal first heart sound is not present. A middiastolic rumble with a presystolic accentuation may be heard at the apex with the bell held lightly. An early diastolic sound resulting from the tumor striking the heart wall may be heard and is similar in timing to the opening snap of mitral stenosis. If the myxoma extends into the left ventricle, a systolic murmur similar to that of mitral regurgitation also may be heard. This latter murmur is heard best at the apex with the diaphragm pressed firmly.

❖ Listen now to a patient with a left atrial myxoma.

A myxoma in the right atrium produces a loud, early systolic sound usually regarded as a wide split first sound, which is heard best with the diaphragm at the left lateral sternal border. It also produces a pulmonic ejection murmur, which is heard best at base left. If the tumor extends into the right ventricle, a systolic murmur similar to that of tricuspid regurgitation also may be heard. This latter murmur is heard best at the left lateral sternal border, with the diaphragm firmly pressed.

Myxomas of the ventricles are rare. If they occur in the right ventricle, the murmur of pulmonic stenosis may be mimicked. A myxoma in the left ventricle would have an auscultatory murmur that mimics aortic stenosis.

## STERNAL CLICK

After heart surgery requiring a median sternotomy, the sternum is assessed daily for signs of instability. One such sign is a **sternal click,** which is audible without a stethoscope when firm pressure is applied along the entire sternum with the fingertips. The presence of a "click" is indicative of sternal bone dehiscence, which is considered a warning sign of sternal infection. The "click" is thought to be produced by sternal-bone–to–sternal-bone motion. Having the patient cough while you apply sternal pressure will accentuate any instability.

## SUBCUTANEOUS EMPHYSEMA

**Subcutaneous emphysema,** the presence of air or gas in the subcutaneous tissues, may be discerned with either palpation or auscultation. The area may appear puffy, and with slight pressure a "crackling" sound (crepitation) may be heard. The sound may be audible with or without the stethoscope over the area. It may occur when air escapes from a tracheostomy or thoracic incision and the air moves under the skin. The air may accumulate around the face, neck and throat, or thorax.

When subcutaneous emphysema occurs over the left chest, the crepitation should be recognized as a noncardiac sound. Generally, subcutaneous emphysema is not serious because the air is eventually reabsorbed by the body.

Its origin also may be a result of infection by gas-producing organisms, especially *Clostridium perfringens*. In the latter case the puffiness and crepitation would appear in the area of the infection.

## MEDIASTINAL CRUNCH

**Mediastinal crunch** is the presence of air in the mediastinum that produces a series of scratchy sounds, which correlate to either respiration or heart beat, but in a random fashion. The discovery of subcutaneous emphysema would confirm the presence of mediastinal crunch. These sounds commonly occur after cardiac surgery. A stethoscope usually is needed to hear them, although the patient may be aware of them.

## ☰  SELF-LEARNING "UNKNOWN" HEART SOUNDS

❖ On the audio program, listen to the "unknown" heart sound and identify the sound. Compare your answers with the answer key at the end of the chapter. Relisten to the audio program as needed to achieve mastery of the content.

1. Is the sound heard a pericardial friction rub, a paradoxical split second sound, a pericardial knock, or a left atrial myxoma?

2. Is the sound heard a left atrial myxoma, a pericardial friction rub, a pericardial knock, or a paradoxical split second sound?

3. Is the sound heard a paradoxical split second sound, a left atrial myxoma, a pericardial knock, or a pericardial friction rub?

4. Is the sound heard a pericardial friction rub, a paradoxical split second sound, a left atrial myxoma, or a pericardial knock?

## ☰  SELF-LEARNING QUESTIONS

Select the letter of the correct response or provide requested information. Compare your answers with the answer key at the end of the chapter. Reread the chapter as needed to achieve mastery of the content.

1. An endocardial pacemaker causes
   a. physiological split of second sound
   b. paradoxical split of second sound
   c. split of first sound
   d. louder-than-normal first sound

2. The etiological factor of a pericardial knock is
   a. constrictive pericarditis
   b. congestive heart failure
   c. uremic pericarditis
   d. none of the above

3. A sternal click is a sign of
   a. mitral valve prolapse
   b. constrictive pericarditis
   c. unstable sternum
   d. subcutaneous emphysema

4. The sound heard when auscultating over subcutaneous emphysema is described as
   a. crackling
   b. click
   c. rub
   d. scratchy

5. The sound heard when auscultating over the presence of air in the mediastinum is described as
   a. crackling
   b. click
   c. rub
   d. scratchy

6. A myxoma in the left atrium has an early diastolic sound similar in timing to the opening snap but is from
   a. mitral regurgitation
   b. mitral stenosis
   c. tumor striking heart wall
   d. tumor extending into left ventricle

## ANSWERS TO SELF-LEARNING "UNKNOWN" HEART SOUNDS

1. Pericardial friction rub

2. Paradoxical split second sound

3. Pericardial knock

4. Left atrial myxoma

## ANSWERS TO SELF-LEARNING QUESTIONS

1. b

2. a

3. c

4. a

5. d

6. c

# *Appendix*

## Chapter 2: The First Heart Sound

Listen now to a sound which is split at various distances. A split of .08 seconds . . . split of .06 seconds . . . split of .04 seconds . . . split of .02 seconds . . . single sound . . . split .02 seconds . . . single sound . . . split .02 seconds . . .

Listen now to a normal heart sound at the various sites. First sound: left lateral sternal border, split . . . first sound: left lateral sternal border, single . . . apex, single first sound . . . base right, single first sound . . . base left, single first sound . . . Intensity of the first sound. Loud sound followed by soft sound . . . soft sound followed by loud sound . . .

Listen to the normal first sound at various sites. Left lateral sternal border, first sound slightly louder than the second sound . . . apex, first sound slightly louder than the second sound . . . base right, first sound slightly softer than the second sound . . .

When listening to a normal first sound, the following is normal for the sites specified: Left lateral sternal border, first sound single slightly louder than the second sound . . . left lateral sternal border, first sound split slightly louder than the second sound . . . apex, first sound single louder than the second . . . base right, first sound single softer than the second . . . base left, first sound single softer than the second . . .

### Self-Learning "Unknown" Heart Sounds—Chapter 2

"Unknown" No. 1 . . .
"Unknown" No. 2 . . .
"Unknown" No. 3 . . .
"Unknown" No. 4 . . .
"Unknown" No. 5 . . .

## Chapter 3: The Second Heart Sound

Listen now to a physiological split second sound. The split is audible on inspiration, the sound single on expiration . . . expiration . . . inspiration . . . expiration . . . inspiration . . . expiration . . . Listen again to a second sound which is split and a second sound which is single. A second sound split . . . a second sound single . . .

Listen now to a normal second sound at the various auscultatory sites: Left lateral sternal border, single second sound . . . apex, single second sound . . . base right, single second sound . . . base left, physiological split second sound . . . inspiration . . . expiration . . . inspiration . . . expiration . . .

Listen to the loudness of the normal second sound at the various auscultatory sites: Left lateral sternal border, second sound softer than the first . . . apex, second sound softer than the first . . . base right, second sound louder than the first . . . base left, second sound louder than the first . . .

When listening to the normal second sound, the following is normal for the sites specified: Left lateral sternal border, second single sound softer than the first . . . apex, second sound single softer than the first . . . base right, second sound single louder than the first . . . base left, second sound splits on inspiration, single on expiration, louder than the first . . . inspiration . . . expiration . . . inspiration . . . expiration . . . inspiration . . . expiration . . .

Review now the normal first and second heart sounds for the sites specified: Left lateral sternal border, single first, single second, first louder than the second . . . left lateral sternal border, split first, single second, first louder than the second . . . apex, single first, single second, first louder than the second . . . base right, single first, single second, first softer than the second . . . base left, single first, physiological split second, first softer than the second . . . inspiration . . . expiration . . . inspiration . . . expiration . . .

**Self-Learning "Unknown" Heart Sounds—Chapter 3**

"Unknown" No. 1 . . . inspiration . . . expiration . . . inspiration . . . expiration . . .
"Unknown" No. 2 . . . inspiration . . . expiration . . . inspiration . . . expiration . . .
"Unknown" No. 3 . . .
"Unknown" No. 4 . . .
"Unknown" No. 5 . . .

## Chapter 4: The Fourth Heart Sound

Listen now to our fourth heart sound. Initially, only $S_1$ and $S_2$ will be heard, then an $S_4$ will be added . . . $S_4$ . . . $S_4$ out . . . $S_4$ . . .

Listen now to a heart with an $S_4$ with a bell lightly held. Then pressure will be put on the bell. Note that the $S_4$ disappears . . . bell lightly held . . . pressure on the bell . . . bell lightly held . . . pressure on the bell . . .

Differentiating $S_4$ from a split first sound . . . listen to an $S_4$ . . . bell lightly held . . . pressure on the bell . . . bell lightly held . . . pressure on the bell . . .

Listen now to a split $S_1$ . . . single first sound . . . split first sound . . . single first sound . . .

Again, listen to an $S_4$ compared to a split $S_1$ . . . $S_4$ . . . . split first
sound . . . single first sound . . . $S_4$ . . . single first sound . . . split first
sound . . . split first sound with an $S_4$ in front of it . . . $S_4$ . . . single first
sound . . . split first sound . . .

**Self-Learning "Unknown" Heart Sounds—Chapter 4**

"Unknown" No. 1: You are listening to the heart at the left lateral sternal border. Using the
   bell lightly held, you hear . . . using the bell firmly pressed, you hear . . . using the
   diaphragm, you hear . . .
"Unknown" No. 2: You are listening to the heart at the left lateral sternal border. Using the
   bell lightly held, you hear . . . using the bell firmly pressed, you hear . . . using the
   diaphragm, you hear . . .
"Unknown" No. 3: You are listening to the heart at the apex. Using the bell lightly held, you
   hear . . . using the bell firmly pressed, you hear . . . using the diaphragm, you hear . . .
"Unknown" No. 4: You are listening to the heart at the apex. Using the bell lightly held, you
   hear . . . using the bell firmly pressed, you hear . . . using the diaphragm, you hear . . .
"Unknown" No. 5: You are listening to the heart at the left lateral sternal border. Using the
   bell lightly held, you hear . . . using the bell firmly pressed, you hear . . . using the
   diaphragm, you hear . . .

# Chapter 5: The Third Heart Sound

Listen now to an $S_3$. Initially, only $S_1$ and $S_2$ will be heard, then $S_3$ will be
added . . . $S_3$ . . . $S_1, S_2$ . . . $S_3$ . . .
Differentiating $S_3$ from $S_4$. Timing permits the $S_3$ to be distinguished from
the $S_4$. $S_3$ comes after the $S_2$ . . . $S_4$ comes before the $S_1$ . . . single $S_1$ and
$S_2$ . . . Listen again: $S_3$ after $S_2$ . . . $S_4$ before $S_1$ . . . single $S_4$ and $S_2$ . . .
quadruple rhythm, $S_4$ in front of $S_1$, $S_3$ after $S_2$ . . . $S_4$ out . . . $S_3$ out . . .
$S_4$ before $S_1$ . . . $S_3$ after $S_2$ . . . summation gallop, $S_3$ and $S_4$ at a rapid
rate . . . $S_3$ and $S_4$ out . . . $S_3$ and $S_4$ in . . . $S_3$ and $S_4$ out . . . $S_3$ and $S_4$
in . . .

**Self-Learning "Unknown" Heart Sounds—Chapter 5**

"Unknown" No. 1: You are listening to the heart at the apex. Using the bell lightly held, you
   hear . . . using the bell firmly pressed, you hear . . . using the diaphragm, you hear . . .
"Unknown" No. 2: You are listening to the heart at base left during inspiration. Using the bell
   lightly held, you hear . . . using the bell firmly pressed, you hear . . . using the
   diaphragm, you hear . . .
"Unknown" No. 3: You are listening to the heart at the apex. Using the bell lightly held, you
   hear . . . using the bell firmly pressed, you hear . . . using the diaphragm, you hear . . .
"Unknown" No. 4: You are listening to the heart at the apex. Using the bell lightly held, you
   hear . . . using the bell firmly pressed, you hear . . . using the diaphragm, you hear . . .
"Unknown" No. 5: You are listening to the heart at the apex. Using the bell lightly held, you
   hear . . . using the bell firmly pressed, you hear . . . using the diaphragm, you hear . . .

## Chapter 6: Murmurs—General Information

Listen now to murmurs that are considered high, medium, and low in frequency, heard equally well with either bell or diaphragm . . . low frequency, heard best with the bell lightly held . . .

Listen now to murmurs that are described as "blowing," "harsh" or "rough," and "rumble." First, listen to a blowing murmur, mainly high frequency . . . now a harsh or rough murmur, mainly medium frequencies . . . now a rumble, mainly low frequencies . . .

Listen now to a heart beating 60 times per minute. First, a systolic blow murmur will be added, then removed . . . systolic blow . . . systolic blow gone . . . systolic blow . . . systolic blow gone . . .*

Listen now to a diastolic rumble. It will be added and removed . . . diastolic rumble . . . diastolic rumble gone . . . diastolic rumble . . . diastolic rumble gone . . .

Listen now to a heart beating 60 times per minute. Then a murmur will be added in the systolic period, early, mid, late, and pan. Early systolic murmur . . . midsystolic murmur . . . late systolic murmur . . . pansystolic murmur . . .

Listen now to a heart beating 60 times per minute. Then a murmur will be added in the diastolic period, early, mid, late, and pandiastolic. First, an early diastolic . . . middiastolic murmur . . . late diastolic murmur . . . pandiastolic murmur . . .

### Self-Learning "Unknown" Heart Sounds—Chapter 6

Determine the frequency of the following sustained sounds:
  "Unknown" No. 1: This sound is heard best with the diaphragm firmly pressed . . .
  "Unknown" No. 2: This sound is heard equally well with either the bell or the diaphragm . . .
  "Unknown" No. 3: This sound is heard best with the bell lightly held . . .
  "Unknown" No. 4: This sound is heard best with the diaphragm firmly pressed . . .
  "Unknown" No. 5: This sound is heard best with the bell lightly held . . .

## Chapter 7: Systolic Murmurs

Listen now to a heart beating 60 times per minute. Then an early systolic murmur will be added . . .

Listen now to a heart beating 60 times per minute. Then an early innocent murmur will be added. The early murmur will then be compared to the one that is midsystolic in type . . . early . . . mid . . .

Listen now to a heart beating 60 times per minute. Then a midsystolic murmur will be added, which is medium in frequency and harsh in quality . . .

*If you are listening to the audio cassette, this is the end of Side A. Please turn over the cassette and continue listening on Side B.

Listen now to a heart beating 60 times per minute. Then a late systolic murmur will be added, which is high in frequency, blowing in quality . . .

Listen now to a heart beating 60 times per minute. Then a pansystolic or holosystolic murmur will be added, which is high in frequency and blowing in quality . . .

**Self-Learning "Unknown" Heart Sounds—Chapter 7**

"Unknown" No. 1 . . .
"Unknown" No. 2 . . .
"Unknown" No. 3 . . .
"Unknown" No. 4 . . .
"Unknown" No. 5 . . .

## Chapter 8: Diastolic Murmurs

Listen now to a heart beating 60 times per minute. Then an early diastolic murmur will be added, which is high in frequency and blowing in quality . . .

Listen now to a heart beating 60 times per minute. Then a middiastolic murmur will be added, which is low in frequency and rumbling in quality . . .

Listen now to a heart beating 60 times per minute. Then a late diastolic murmur will be added, which is low in frequency and rumbling in quality . . .

Listen now to a heart beating 60 times per minute. Then a pandiastolic murmur is added, which is low in frequency and rumbling in quality . . .

**Self-Learning "Unknown" Heart Sounds—Chapter 8**

Listen to the following diastolic murmurs:
  "Unknown" No. 1 . . .
  "Unknown" No. 2 . . .
  "Unknown" No. 3 . . .
  "Unknown" No. 4 . . .
  "Unknown" No. 5 . . .

## Chapter 9: Sounds Around the First Sound

Listen to a wide split first sound as compared with a normal split first sound and a single first sound . . . single first sound . . . wide split first sound . . . single first sound . . . normal split first sound . . . single first sound . . . normal split first sound . . . wide split first sound . . . single first sound . . . normal split first sound . . . wide split first sound . . .

### *Pulmonic Ejection Sounds:*
Pulmonic ejection sound compared to the single first sound . . . single first sound . . . pulmonic ejection sound . . . single first sound . . . pulmonic ejection sound . . .

### *Aortic Ejection Sounds:*

Aortic ejection sound compared to single first sounds . . . single first sound . . . aortic ejection sounds . . . single first sound . . . aortic ejection sound . . .

### *Midsystolic Clicks:*

Midsystolic click compared to single first sound . . . single first sound . . . midsystolic click . . . single first sound . . . midsystolic click . . .

A midsystolic click will move closer to the first sound with standing . . . midsystolic click . . . standing . . . single first sound . . . midsystolic click . . . standing . . .

A midsystolic click will move farther from the first sound with squatting . . . midsystolic click . . . squatting . . . single first sound . . . midsystolic click . . . squatting . . .

### Self-Learning "Unknown" Heart Sounds—Chapter 9

"Unknown" No. 1: You are listening to the heart at base left, with the diaphragm firmly pressed.

"Unknown" No. 2: You are listening to a heart with the diaphragm firmly pressed at the left lateral sternal border, you hear . . . at the apex, you hear . . . at base right, you hear . . . at base left, you hear . . .

"Unknown" No. 3: You are listening to a heart with the diaphragm firmly pressed. At the left lateral sternal border, you hear . . . at the apex, you hear . . . at base right, you hear . . . at base left, you hear . . .

"Unknown" No. 4: You are listening to a heart with the diaphragm firmly pressed. At the left lateral sternal border, you hear . . . at the apex, you hear . . . at base right, you hear . . . at base left, you hear . . .

"Unknown" No. 5: You are listening to the heart at the apex. Using the bell lightly held, you hear . . . using the bell firmly pressed, you hear . . . using the diaphragm, you hear . . .

## Chapter 10: Sounds Around the Second Sound

Listen now to a paradoxical second sound. The split is audible on expiration. The sound is single on inspiration . . . expiration . . . inspiration . . . expiration . . . inspiration . . .

Listen now to a wide split second compared to a single second sound . . . wide split second sound . . . normal split second sound . . . single second sound . . . wide split second sound . . . normal split second sound . . . single second sound . . .

Listen now to a fixed split second sound . . . fixed split second sound . . . inspiration . . . expiration . . . physiological split second sound . . . inspiration . . . expiration . . . inspiration . . . expiration . . .

Listen now to a narrow split second compared to a physiological split second . . . narrow split second sound . . . inspiration . . . expiration . . . inspiration . . . expiration . . . physiological split second sound . . . inspiration . . . expiration . . . inspiration . . . expiration . . .

Listen now to a second sound followed by an opening snap. The opening snap will be taken in and out . . . opening snap present . . . opening snap gone . . . opening snap present . . . opening snap gone . . .

Differentiating $S_3$ from the opening snap. First an opening snap will be heard . . . opening snap gone . . . $S_3$ . . . $S_3$ gone . . . opening snap . . . opening snap gone . . . $S_3$ . . . $S_3$ gone . . . opening snap . . . followed by $S_3$ . . .

### Self-Learning "Unknown" Heart Sounds—Chapter 10

You are listening to the heart at base left, with the diaphragm firmly pressed.
  "Unknown" No. 1 . . . inspiration . . . expiration . . . inspiration . . . expiration . . . inspiration . . . expiration . . .
  "Unknown" No. 2 . . . inspiration . . . expiration . . . inspiration . . . expiration . . . inspiration . . . expiration . . .
  "Unknown" No. 3 . . .
  "Unknown" No. 4: You are listening to the heart at the apex. Using the bell lightly held, you hear . . . using the bell firmly pressed, you hear . . . using the diaphragm firmly pressed, you hear . . .
  "Unknown" No. 5: You are listening to the heart at the apex. Using the bell lightly held, you hear . . . using the bell firmly pressed, you hear . . . using the diaphragm firmly pressed, you hear . . .

## Chapter 11: Friction Rubs—Pericardial and Pleural

Listen now to a pericardial friction rub at the rate of 60 with both systolic and diastolic sounds . . .

Listen to a heart beating 60 times per minute, then only the systolic component of the rub will be added . . .

Listen to a heart beating 60 times per minute, then only the diastolic components of the rub will be added . . .

Now listen to a pericardial friction rub at the heart rate of 120 . . .

Listen to a real heart with a pericardial friction rub. All three components are present . . .

Listen now to a pleural friction rub from a real individual. Note the inspiratory/expiratory components . . .

Compare a pleural friction rub to a pericardial friction rub. First a pleural friction rub . . . now a pericardial friction rub . . .

### Self-Learning "Unknown" Heart Sounds—Chapter 11

"Unknown" No. 1: You are listening to the left lateral sternal border. You hear the following sound . . .
"Unknown" No. 2: You are listening to the heart at the apex. You hear the following sound . . .

## Chapter 12: Prosthetic Valve Sounds

Listen now to a patient with a caged-ball valve, the Starr-Edwards . . .

Listen now to a patient with a porcine heart valve in the aortic position . . .

**Self-Learning "Unknown" Heart Sounds—Chapter 12**

"Unknown" No. 1 . . .
"Unknown" No. 2 . . .


## Chapter 13: Sounds Postheart Surgery and Other Sounds

Listen now to a patient with pericardial friction rub . . .

Listen now to a patient with a paradoxical splitting of the second heart sound as heard with an endocardial pacemaker in the right ventricle . . .

Listen now to a patient with a pericardial knock . . .

Listen now to a patient with a left atrial myxoma . . .

**Self-Learning "Unknown" Heart Sounds—Chapter 13**

"Unknown" No. 1 . . .
"Unknown" No. 2 . . .
"Unknown" No. 3 . . .
"Unknown" No. 4 . . .

# Bibliography

Blome-Eberwein SA et al: Impact of mechanical heart valve prosthesis sound on patients' quality of life, *Ann Thorac Surg* 61:594-602, 1996.

Caccamo L, Erickson B: *Cardiac auscultation,* Youngstown, Ohio, 1975, St. Elizabeth Hospital Medical Center.

Carabello BA: *Cardiology clinics: valvular heart disease,* Philadelphia, 1991, WB Saunders.

Constant J: *Bedside cardiology,* Boston, 1969, Little, Brown.

Erickson B: Detecting abnormal heart sounds, *Nurs 86,* 16(1):58-63, 1986.

Erickson RL: An in vitro study of mechanical heart valve sound loudness, *J Heart Valve Dis,* 3(3):330-334, 1994.

Frankl WS, Brest AN: *Valvular heart disease: comprehensive evaluation and treatment, cardiovascular clinics* ed 2, Philadelphia, 1993, FA Davis.

Harris A et al, editors: *Physiological and clinical aspects of cardiac auscultation,* Philadelphia, 1976, JB Lippincott.

Harvey WP, Canfield DC: *Clinical auscultation of the cardiovascular system: tapes with companion tests,* Newton, NJ, 1989, Laennec Publishing.

Vaska PL: Sternal wound infections, *AACN Clinical Issues* 4(3):475-483, 1993.

# Glossary

**A₂:** Aortic component of the second heart sound ($S_2$); normally comes before the pulmonic component ($P_2$).

**Allograft:** Tissue grafts from individuals of the same species (isograft).

**Aortic ejection sound:** *See* Ejection sounds, aortic.

**Aortic valve:** Semilunar valve that prevents the backflow of blood from the aorta into the left ventricle during ventricular diastole. The closure of this valve is responsible for the first component ($A_2$) of the second heart sound.

**Apex:** Area of cardiac auscultation. Also known as the point of maximum impulse (PMI) of the heart against the chest wall. In the normal adult it is at the fifth intercostal space to the left of the sternum at the midclavicular line. Sounds from the mitral valve and the left heart are heard best in this area.

**Atrial kick:** Slang term for atrial systole or atrial contraction that may contribute 20% to 25% to ventricular filling. It occurs during the late filling phase of the ventricular diastolic period but only if atrial contraction occurs. It can never occur in the presence of atrial fibrillation.

**Atrial systole:** *See* Systole, atrial.

**Auscultogram:** A graphic method of charting heart sounds.

**Base left:** Area of cardiac auscultation; the second intercostal space to the left of the sternum. Sounds from the pulmonic valve are heard best in this area.

**Base right:** Area of cardiac auscultation; the second intercostal space to the right of the sternum. Sounds from the aortic valve are heard best in this area.

**Bell chestpiece:** Component of the stethoscope that has a shallow shell with a diameter as large as feasible to permit an air seal when held lightly on the chest wall so that no after-imprint is left. It transmits sounds of **low** frequency.

**Bileaflet:** Type of mechanical prosthetic heart valve with two semicircular leaflets mounted on a circular sewing ring that opens in the center.

**Biological prosthetic heart valve:** A valve made from tissue of the same species (allograft) or from different species (xenograft).

**Bovine pericardial heart valve:** A prosthetic heart valve made from a cow. It consists of three identical cusps mounted on a cloth-covered frame.

**Caged-ball:** Type of mechanical prosthetic heart valve consisting of a ball that moves freely within a three- or four-sided metallic cage mounted on a circular sewing ring.

**Cardiac cycle:** The period from the beginning of one beat of the heart to the beginning of the next succeeding beat; consists of two phases: one of contraction, systole—atrial and ventricular; and one of relaxation, diastole—atrial and ventricular.

**Click:** High-frequency sound that is heard after the first heart sound ($S_1$). It may be a single or multiple sound heard in the middle of ventricular systolic period; often associated with mitral valve prolapse.

**Compliance:** The ratio of change in volume to a change in pressure (V/P). Ventricular compliance is decreased in the presence of any condition that limits the ability of the ventricle(s) to expand. Decreased ventricular compliance is one mechanism responsible for the production of the third ($S_3$) and the fourth ($S_4$) heart sounds.

**Diaphragm chestpiece:** A component of the stethoscope that has a taut (stiff) material drawn across its diameter. When it is firmly applied to the chest wall (leaving an after-imprint), it transmits sounds of **high** frequency.

**Diastole, ventricular:** Period of ventricular filling that follows closure of the aortic and pulmonic valves. The ventricular diastolic period is divided into three phases:
1. The first third of the diastolic period, which has two subdivisions— the isovolumic relaxation phase and the rapid filling phase.
2. The middle third of the diastolic period, during which both atrium and ventricles are relaxed.
3. The last third of diastole, or the late filling phase, during which atrial contraction takes place.

**Diastolic murmurs:** *See* Murmurs, diastolic.

**Duration:** The length of time that a sound lasts. Normal heart sounds ($S_1$ and $S_2$) are of short duration. Cardiac murmurs or rubs are of long duration.

**Ejection murmur:** *See* Murmurs—mid.

**Ejection sounds:** These are high-frequency "clicking" sounds occurring very shortly after the first sound. They may be of either aortic or pulmonic origin.
> **Aortic:** High-frequency "clicking" sound heard best at the apex but may be heard anywhere on a straight line from base right to the apex. Heard in valvular aortic stenosis, aortic insufficiency, coarctation of the aorta, and aneurysm of the ascending aorta.
> **Pulmonic:** High-frequency "clicking" sound heard best at base left but may be heard anywhere along the left lateral sternal border. It may be heard in pulmonic stenosis, pulmonary hypertension, atrial sep-

tal defect, pulmonary embolism, hyperthyroidism, or in conditions causing enlargement of the pulmonary artery.

**First heart sound:** The initial sound heard—also known as $S_1$. It occurs at the beginning of ventricular systole when ventricular volume is maximal. It is a result of the closure of the mitral ($M_1$) and tricuspid ($T_1$) valves.

> **Split, normal:** When both mitral and tricuspid closure are distinguishable and are 0.02 second apart.
>
> **Split, wide:** Mitral and tricuspid closure sounds occur wider apart from either electrical or mechanical causes that result in ventricular asynchrony.

**Fourth heart sound:** The fourth heart sound is a low-frequency sound heard just before the first heart sound. It is a result of decreased ventricular compliance or increased volume of filling. It also is known as an "atrial gallop," "presystolic gallop," "$S_4$ gallop," and "$S_4$."

**Frequency:** The number of wave cycles generated per second by a vibrating body. It is the vibratory movement of an object in motion that initiates the sound wave cycles that can be discerned with the stethoscope.

> **High:** The greater the number of wave cycles per second generated by a vibrating body, the higher the frequency. Sounds of high frequency are heard best with the diaphragm chestpiece firmly pressed.
>
> **Low:** The fewer the number of wave cycles per second generated by a vibrating body, the lower the frequency. Sounds of low frequency are heard best with the bell chestpiece lightly applied.
>
> **Mid:** Combination of high and low frequencies. Sound heard equally well with either bell or diaphragm.

**Heart sound simulator:** An electronic device designed to generate all normal and abnormal heart sound patterns by the independent variation of all sound parameters.

**Heterologous:** Derived from tissue of a different species (xenograft).

**Intensity:** Intensity determines the loudness of the perceived sound. It is related to the height of the sound wave produced by a vibrating object. Objects vibrating with great energy are heard as loud sounds. Objects vibrating with low energy are heard as soft sounds.

**Intraaortic balloon pump:** A mechanical device that aids the heart's circulation through counterpulsation; it expands in diastole and collapses in systole.

**Isograft:** Tissue grafts from individuals of the same species (allograft).

**Isovolumic contraction:** A phase during the first part of ventricular systole. It begins with the first initial rise in ventricular pressure after the closure of the mitral and tricuspid valves.

**Isovolumic relaxation:** A phase during the first third of the ventricular diastole. Initially in this period no blood is entering the ventricles, and the ventricles therefore are not increasing in volume.

**Late filling phase:** A phase during the last third of ventricular diastole. It is at this time that the "atrial kick" or atrial contraction takes place.

**Left lateral recumbent:** Position for cardiac auscultation in which the patient is lying on his/her left side with left arm extended under head. The heart is brought closer to the chest wall in this position. Also the exertion of turning to this position increases heart rate. This position may be useful in making audible the diastolic rumble of mitral stenosis, the low-frequency third heart sound ($S_3$) of congestive heart failure.

**Left lateral sternal border:** Area of cardiac auscultation that is at the left fourth intercostal space to the left of the sternum. Sounds from the tricuspid valve and right heart are heard best in this area.

**$M_1$:** The mitral component of the first heart sound. This is normally the first component and occurs just after the mitral valve closes; normally comes before the tricuspid component ($T_1$).

**Mechanical prosthetic heart valve:** A type of prosthetic heart valve made from a combination of metal alloys, pyrolyte carbon, and Dacron.

**Mediastinal crunch:** Presence of air in the mediastinum that produces a series of scratchy sounds.

**Mitral valve:** Bicuspid valve between the left atrium and the left ventricle; one of two "A-V" valves; prevents backflow of blood from left ventricle to left atrium during ventricular systole. Closure of this valve is responsible for the first component ($M_1$) of the first heart sound.

**Mitral valve prolapse:** Syndrome associated with a midsystolic click and a late systolic murmur. One of the mitral leaflets, usually the posterior one, balloons into the left atrium at the point of maximal ventricular ejection. The click is heard when the chordae tendineae suddenly stop the ballooning leaflet. If the leaflets pull apart, a late systolic murmur of mitral regurgitation also may be heard. Also known as "Barlow's syndrome," "floppy mitral valve," or "click-murmur syndrome."

**Murmurs:** Sustained noises that are audible during the time periods of systole, diastole, or both.

  **Diastolic murmurs:** Sustained noises that are audible between the second heart sound and the next first heart sound. They should be considered organic and not normal. Common causes include mitral or tricuspid stenosis and aortic or pulmonic regurgitation.

  **Early:** Peaks in the first third of the cycle.

  **Late:** Peaks in the later third of the cycle.

  **Mid:** Peaks in the middle of the cycle; "crescendo/decrescendo" (diamond shaped). Also known as "ejection" murmur.

  **Pan:** Heard continuously throughout the cycle.

  **Systolic murmurs:** Sustained noises that are audible between the first and the second heart sounds. Common causes include mitral or tricuspid regurgitation and aortic or pulmonic stenosis.

**Myxoma:** A soft tumor primarily composed of connective tissue.

**Opening snap:** Short, high-frequency "click" or "snap" that occurs after the second heart sound. It is most often produced by the opening of a stenosed, thickened, or distorted mitral or tricuspid valve.

**$P_2$:** Pulmonic component of the second heart sound; usually follows aortic component ($A_2$).

**Pacemaker:** An electrical apparatus used to electrically stimulate the heart and regulate the heart beat.

**Pericardial knock:** An early diastolic sound occurring in constrictive pericarditis.

**Pitch:** Subjective sensation that indicates to the listener whether the tone is high or low on a musical scale.

**Point of maximal impulse:** Area on the chest at which the heart is best palpable; usually corresponds to apex, which in a normal adult is located at the fifth intercostal space, midclavicular line, to the left of the sternum.

**Porcine heart valve:** A prosthetic heart valve made from a pig. It is mounted on a semiflexible stent and preserved with glutaraldehyde.

**Prosthetic heart valve:** An artificial valve, either mechanical or biological, used to replace a damaged heart valve.

**Pulmonic ejection sound:** *See* Ejection sounds, pulmonic.

**Pulmonic valve:** Semilunar valve that prevents backflow of blood from the pulmonary artery into the right ventricle during ventricular diastole. Closure of the valve is responsible for the second component ($P_2$) of the second heart sound.

**Quality:** This is a sound characteristic that distinguishes two sounds that have equal degrees of frequency and intensity but come from a different source—e.g., piano from a violin, or heart from lung.

   **Blow:** Mainly high frequency.

   **Harsh:** Mix of high and low frequencies—slightly more high than low.

   **Rough:** Mix of high and low frequencies—slightly more low than high.

   **Rumble:** Mainly low frequency.

**Rapid filling phase:** Phase during the first third of ventricular diastole. It occurs when ventricular pressure is less than atrial pressure. The mitral and tricuspid valves then open and blood rapidly enters the ventricles.

**Rapid ventricular ejection:** Phase during the first part of ventricular systole. It follows the isovolumic contraction phase. It occurs when ventricular pressure exceeds the pressure in the aorta and the pulmonary artery, forcing the aortic and pulmonic valves open and causing blood to be rapidly ejected from the ventricles.

**$S_1$:** *See* First heart sound.

**$S_2$:** *See* Second heart sound.

**$S_3$:** *See* Third heart sound.

**$S_4$:** *See* Fourth heart sound.

**Second heart sound:** Second sound heard in a normal heart—also known as $S_2$. It occurs at the end of ventricular systole. It is a result of the closure of the aortic ($A_2$) and pulmonic ($P_2$) valves.

**Split, fixed:** This split does not change its width with inspiration or expiration.

**Split, narrow:** The aortic ($A_2$) and pulmonic ($P_2$) components are closer together than normal—<0.03 second. The split is heard on **inspiration** and is single on expiration.

**Split, paradoxical:** Reversal of the normal closure sequence of $S_2$, with pulmonic closure ($P_2$) occurring before aortic closure ($A_2$). This split is heard during **expiration** and becomes single on inspiration. (The opposite of a normal or physiological split.)

**Split, physiological:** The aortic ($A_2$) and pulmonic ($P_2$) components that make up the second sound are separately distinguishable—0.03 second apart. The split is heard on **inspiration** and is single on expiration.

**Split, wide:** Delay in pulmonic valve closure can cause the physiological split to be accentuated or increased—0.04 to 0.05 second. The split is heard during **inspiration** and becomes single on expiration.

**Sine wave:** An up and down or to and fro undulating or wavy line.

**Split:** When both components that make up a sound are separately distinguishable, the sound is said to "split." A duration of 0.02 second between the sounds is necessary for the ear to be able to make this distinction. See first sound, split and/or second sound, split.

**Sternum, unstable:** Indicative of sternal dehiscence after a median sternotomy. Sternal click is a sign of instability.

**Stethoscope:** Acoustical instrument that uses the vibration of sounds reacting on the air column enclosed in tubing to transmit sounds to the listener's ear. When used for heart sounds, a bell and diaphragm chestpiece are necessary.

**Subcutaneous emphysema:** The presence of air or gas in the subcutaneous tissues.

**Systole, atrial:** Period in cardiac cycle. It occurs during the last third of ventricular diastole or during the late filling phase. During this period contraction of the atrium takes place and the remaining blood is squeezed from the atrium. This also is known as the "atrial kick." Atrial systole may contribute 20% to 25% to ventricular filling. The contribution is less at faster heart rates—greater than 100 beats per minute.

**Systole, ventricular:** Period in cardiac cycle. It follows closure of the mitral and tricuspid valves. This systolic period is divided into two phases: (1) The first phase includes the isovolumic contraction phase and the rapid ventricular ejection phase. (2) During the latter part of ventricular systole, ventricular pressure falls, and reduced ventricular ejection occurs. This period lasts until ventricular ejection stops and ventricular diastole begins.

**Systolic murmurs:** *See* Murmurs, systolic.

**$T_1$:** Second component of the first sound. It normally occurs after $M_1$ (the mitral component) just after the tricuspid valve closes.

**Third heart sound:** Low-frequency sound heard just after the second heart sound. It is a diastolic sound that occurs during the early rapid filling phase of ventricular diastole. It is a result of decreased ventricular compliance or increased ventricular diastolic volume. It also is known as a "ventricular gallop," "protodiastolic gallop," "$S_3$ gallop," or "$S_3$."

**Thrill:** Continuous palpable sensation felt on the precordium. It is comparable to the vibration felt when a cat purrs.

**Thrust:** Palpable (sometimes even visible) intermittent sensation. This is the sensation felt when palpating the point of maximal impulse (PMI) at the apex of the heart.

**Tilting disk:** A type of mechanical valve with a free-floating, lens-shaped disk mounted on a circular sewing ring.

**Timing:** Determining whether sound is occurring during the systolic or diastolic period.

**Timing, finer:** Determining whether sound is occurring early, mid, late, or pan in the systolic or diastolic period.

**Tricuspid valve:** Three-leaflet valve between the right atrium and the right ventricle: one of two A-V valves; prevents backflow of blood from the right ventricle to right atrium during ventricular systole. Closure of this valve is responsible for the second component ($T_1$) of the first heart sound.

**Turbulence:** Smooth blood flow is disturbed, and the blood flows crosswise in the vessel or chamber, as well as along the vessel. This causes eddy currents similar to a whirlpool and produces vibrations that are audible.

**Ventricular diastole:** *See* Diastole, ventricular.

**Ventricular systole:** *See* Systole, ventricular.

**Xenograft:** Derived from tissue of a different species (heterologous).

# Index

A

A$_2$; *see* Aortic closure

A$_1$ component of second heart sound; *see* Aortic component of second heart sound

Acceleration of blood, cardiac sound production and, 8-9

Adipose tissue, increased, sound transmission and, 10

Age, perception of sounds and, 11

Air, sound transmission and, 10

Air-trapping, sound transmission and, 10

Allograft biological heart valves, 93

Amplifying stethoscopes, 11

Amyl nitrate, inhalation of, murmurs and, 52

Anemia

  first heart sound and, 25

  S$_4$ of left ventricular origin and, 36

Aneurysm

  aortic, aortic regurgitation and, 65

  of ascending aorta, aortic ejection sounds and, 69

  Anterior-posterior (A-P) diameter, sound transmission and, 10

Aorta

  ascending, aneurysm of, aortic ejection sounds and, 69

  coarctation of, aortic ejection sounds and, 69

Aortic aneurysm, aortic regurgitation and, 65

Aortic area, auscultation and, 5

Aortic closure (A$_2$)

  paradoxical split S$_2$ and, 76

  second heart sound and, 30

Aortic (A$_1$) component of second heart sound, 22

Aortic diastolic murmurs, 64-65

Aortic ejection sounds, 69

  audio program for, 108

Aortic insufficiency

  aortic ejection sounds and, 69

  first heart sound and, 25

Aortic regurgitation

  diastolic murmurs and, 51, 63, 64-65

  early diastolic murmurs and, 62

  hand-grip maneuver and, 52

  paradoxical split S$_2$ and, 76

  uncomplicated patent ductus arteriosus with, narrow split S$_2$ and, 78

Aortic stenosis

  amyl nitrate and, 52

  hand-grip maneuver and, 52

  left ventricular myxomas and, 100

  midsystolic murmurs and, 57

  narrow split S$_2$ and, 78

  paradoxical split S$_2$ and, 76

  S$_4$ of left ventricular origin and, 36, 38

  systolic murmurs and, 51, 56, 58, 59

  valvular, aortic ejection sounds and, 69

Aortic valve

  auscultation and, 5

  sounds of, 8

Aortic valve incompetence, diastolic murmurs and, 62

A-P diameter; *see* Anterior-posterior diameter

Apex, auscultation and, 5

Ascending aorta, aneurysm of, aortic ejection sounds and, 69

Atrial contraction, cardiac cycle and, 7

Atrial fibrillation

  absence of fourth heart sound in, 38

  fourth heart sound and, 36

Atrial gallop, 36; *see also* Fourth heart sound

Atrial kick, 7

  fourth heart sound and, 36

Atrial septal defect

  fixed split S$_2$ and, 78

  opening snap and, 79

  pulmonic ejection sounds and, 69

  wide split S$_2$ and, 77

Atrial systole, 7

Audio program, transcript for, 103-110

Auscultation

  areas of, 4-5

  father of, 2

  history of, 2

  pericardial friction rubs and, 84

  pleural friction rubs and, 84

  requirements for, 2-6

  selective listening and, 5-6